Nature's Pharmacy

The Art of Healing at Home

By

Elara Greenwood

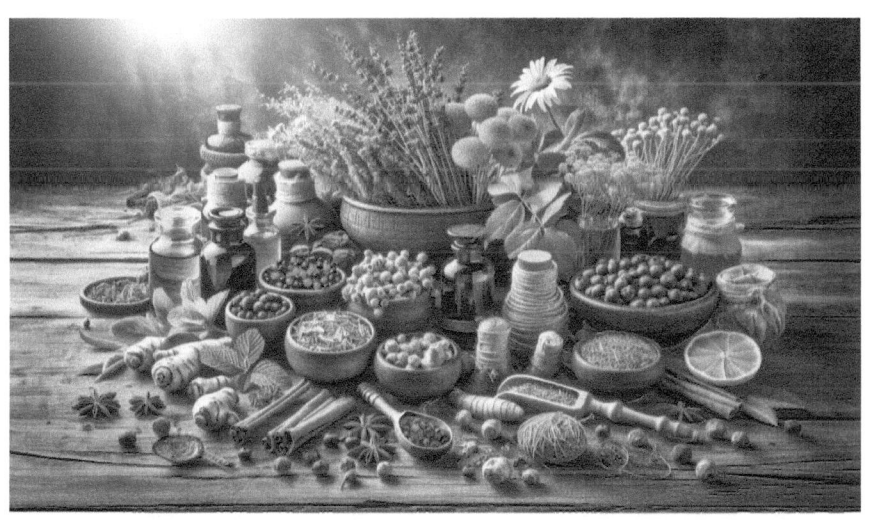

Table of Contents

Introduction

In a world that's increasingly turning back to nature for solutions, the quest for health and wellness through home-based remedies has become more relevant than ever. This shift is driven by a desire to step away from conventional pharmaceuticals and their potential side effects, and instead, embrace the holistic healing power offered by nature. Whether it's a soothing cup of chamomile tea to calm a restless mind or a dash of turmeric to add vibrancy and vitality to your meals, natural remedies have found their way into the routines of many health-conscious individuals.

The concept of healing is as ancient as humankind itself. Our ancestors, seeking to understand the mysteries of health and sickness, turned to their surroundings for answers. Plants, herbs, and natural compounds were not just resources for survival; they became the foundation of early medicine. By observing and experimenting, ancient civilizations like the Egyptians, Chinese, and Greeks learned the art of utilizing nature's bounty to promote healing and wellness. These practices have evolved, and today, we're rediscovering and validating them through modern insights and scientific research.

Home remedies aren't merely alternative solutions; they represent a lifestyle choice that's deeply rooted in tradition and sustainability. As the world becomes more aware of health and environmental issues, this approach offers a harmonious blend of simplicity and efficacy. It's not about rejecting modern medicine altogether; rather, it's about complementing it—bridging the gap between ancient wisdom and modern science. This book aims to guide you on this journey towards balance, ensuring your path is informed, effective, and empathetic to your unique needs.

Everyone's path to wellness is individual, and so must be their approach to using natural remedies. What works for one might not work for another, and that's the beauty of nature's versatility. Through understanding various home remedies, you gain the ability to choose what resonates with your body and spirit. This book is not just a compiled list of remedies; it's a gateway to empowering yourself with knowledge and resources to sustain a healthy lifestyle.

Why, you might ask, should one turn to home remedies? The answer lies in accessibility, affordability, and self-sufficiency. Many remedies can be found right in your kitchen cupboard or garden, easily accessible for immediate use. The power to heal, soothe, and rejuvenate is right at your fingertips, waiting to be unlocked. You save not only money but also gain greater control over what goes into your body, fostering a personal connection to your health care.

Moreover, the practice of preparing your own remedies can be profoundly therapeutic. There's a certain satisfaction in knowing what you're using has been crafted by your own hands, with intention and care. Whether it's mixing a balm for sore muscles or brewing a tea for a sore throat, these practices invite mindfulness into daily routines, enhancing both mental and physical well-being.

For many, the reliance on pharmaceuticals is not merely a preference but a necessity. These remedies shouldn't be seen as replacements for essential medicines but as complementary practices that can enhance one's overall health. When integrated mindfully, they can help reduce reliance on medications, address minor ailments, and improve general well-being through prevention and holistic care.

Through the pages that follow, you'll find a rich tapestry of techniques and knowledge that span across centuries and cultures.

Each chapter delves into a specific aspect of natural healing—from herbal medicine and essential oils to nutrition and homeopathy—providing you with the insights needed to embrace this way of life. The guidance offered here is both practical and inspirational, encouraging you to explore and adapt these practices into your everyday living.

Our collective journey will not stop at physical health. The mind-body connection, an integral part of natural healing, will weave through the chapters, urging you to consider wellness in a holistic sense. Practices such as mindfulness and meditation are essential companions on this journey, showcasing how emotional and mental well-being are deeply intertwined with physical health.

The landscape of home remedies is as broad and diverse as the earth itself, waiting to be explored, understood, and cherished. It's an invitation to discover your own rhythm of life through nature's timeless gifts. With an open heart and inquisitive mind, you'll find your path to health is not just about alleviating symptoms but about cultivating a life that's vibrant, balanced, and in harmony with the world around you.

This book serves as a roadmap for those seeking a deeper connection with their health and well-being, offering not only remedies but a philosophy that appreciates the intricate dance between environment and evolution. Each remedy and practice shared herein speaks of a heritage worth preserving and a knowledge that empowers you to take health into your own hands. Let's embark on this empowering journey towards natural healing, unlocking the innate wisdom that lies within us all.

Chapter 1:
The History of Home Remedies

Home remedies have woven themselves into the fabric of human history, offering a tapestry of healing practices passed down through generations. From the ancient wisdom of herbal brews to age-old acupuncture techniques, these remedies have been our ancestors' trusted companions in nurturing health. They tell stories of survival and adaptation, where early civilizations relied on their intimate knowledge of plants, minerals, and simple rituals to stave off ailments. As modern medicine emerged, home remedies didn't vanish; instead, they evolved, harmonizing age-old traditions with contemporary insights. This blending of the past and present provides a gentle reminder that the pursuit of wellness is a timeless endeavor, accessible to anyone willing to embrace the natural world. Restoring balance through these remedies promises not just relief but empowerment, an invitation to actively participate in one's health journey. As we explore the origins and evolution of these practices, we uncover the profound impact they can have on our lives today.

Origins of Natural Healing

The history of natural healing traces a path as old as humanity itself. From the dawn of civilization, people turned to nature to heal and nourish their bodies. The whisper of leaves, the quiet rustle of herbs, and the invigorating scent of spices comprise the ancient tapestry that continues to impact our lives today. Before the advent of modern medicine, every culture cultivated its own repertoire of healing practices, deeply rooted in the natural world surrounding them.

It's fascinating to consider how these early societies experimented with native plants, learning through trial and observation which herbs held the power to heal or which plants could soothe a persistent ailment. This proto-science was based on deep observation, a respect for nature, and an understanding that the body has inherent healing capabilities. For many, natural healing wasn't just a way to treat disease; it was an integral part of daily life and survival.

Have you ever wondered how treatments were shared across different cultures? Ancient traders and travelers played a crucial role in exchanging knowledge of natural medicines. Think of them as the original natural medicine carriers, sharing seeds, roots, and stories as they journeyed from one land to another. Along the Silk Road, for instance, they didn't just trade silk and spices; they exchanged medicinal herbs and healing wisdom that enriched diverse cultures along the way.

In Ancient Egypt, the healing arts were advanced, with papyrus scrolls revealing some of the earliest known medical documentation. Egyptian healers blended spirituality and science in their treatments, employing a variety of plants and minerals. Many of the herbs they used, like fennel and garlic, are still valued in modern herbal medicine for their potent health benefits. Their approaches laid the groundwork for subsequent cultures, including the Greeks and Romans, who wove these practices into their own medical frameworks.

The Greeks were pioneers in recognizing the importance of balance for overall well-being, a principle that echoes across the ages in healing disciplines. Hippocrates, often hailed as the "Father of Medicine," believed in treating the whole patient, not just the symptoms, and he sought to harness nature's power in the healing process. His renowned aphorism, "Let food be thy medicine," captures the essence of using natural means to support the body's health.

Entirely different yet beautifully aligned, Traditional Chinese Medicine (TCM) also emerged as a sophisticated system over 2,000 years ago. Rooted in the philosophy of harmony between mind, body, and environment, TCM emphasizes the vital life force or "Qi". This ancient approach incorporates herbs, acupuncture, and dietary practices to maintain this delicate balance. Once regarded as mystical, many TCM practices are now scientifically recognized for their efficacy in promoting health and preventing disease.

In the Americas, indigenous cultures developed rich traditions that relied on the local flora for healing. Plants like echinacea and ginseng were not only vital for remedying ailments but were revered for their spiritual significance as well. Native healers approached illness by seeking balance within not just the body, but the entire universe, cultivating a profound respect for the interconnectedness of all life.

Ayurveda, with its roots deeply entrenched in the Indian subcontinent, offers another ancient holistic system of medicine. Emphasizing balance among body, mind, and spirit—as well as harmony with the environment—its principles of diet, herbs, and lifestyle have provided a framework for health that remains tremendously influential. Ayurveda considers that health is the outcome of a harmony between oneself and the universe, which guides its approach to treatment and prevention.

The natural healing traditions across the world underscore a shared understanding that nature holds the key to health and vitality. Though each culture adapted these practices in unique ways, they all gravitated towards a central belief—healing is most effective when it works in harmony with nature. As people discovered what plants and herbs could do, they documented their properties, passed their knowledge through generations, and crafted remedies that have stood the test of time.

Today, as modern medicine continues to evolve, there's a growing acknowledgement of the value of ancient wisdom. Natural healing, with its emphasis on prevention, holistic treatment, and mindfulness, complements conventional approaches by empowering individuals to participate actively in their wellness. Instead of focusing solely on symptoms, it encourages a deeper understanding of one's body and its innate ability to heal.

This revival rests not on a rejection of modern advancements but on an integrated approach—one that merges the wisdom of the past with the innovation of the present. The roots of natural healing run deep, reminding us that even in an era dominated by pharmaceuticals, the gifts of nature remain an enduring source of health and hope.

As we reconnect with these ancient practices, we not only honor the legacy of those who walked before us but also pave the way for a future where the harmony between humanity and nature is restored. In turning to the origins of natural healing, we are reminded of the beauty, power, and wisdom inherent in the world around us. Embracing this knowledge, we're inspired to explore, adapt, and find our unique path towards wellness, deeply aware that the answers to many of our modern health challenges lie in the oldest of traditions.

Traditional Practices and Modern Insights

Throughout history, home remedies have stood as a testament to human ingenuity and resilience. Long before the pharmaceutical giants dominated the health landscape, individuals relied on what nature provided—from herbs and plants to minerals and the elements. While the traditions vary globally, the essence of natural healing has remained consistent: to harness the inherent power of the earth to restore balance and health. Our ancestors may not have possessed today's scientific tools, but they had something equally powerful—centuries of accumulated wisdom.

It's fascinating to observe the role of ancient practices in today's health revolution. With the vast knowledge at our disposal, one might assume we'd have left traditional remedies in the past. Yet, the opposite seems to be true. As people across the globe seek to reduce their dependency on synthetic medications, there's a renewed interest in the efficacy and simplicity of age-old healing methods. This fusion of traditional practices with modern insights is creating a robust dialogue between the past and the present, encouraging us to relearn what was once common knowledge.

In many cultures, traditional medicine is still the primary modality. Take Ayurveda from India or Traditional Chinese Medicine; both have histories spanning thousands of years, and both integrate a comprehensive understanding of the human body with the healing powers of nature. Modern research is not only validating the effectiveness of some of these treatments but also providing insights into how and why they work. For instance, curcumin, the active ingredient in turmeric—a staple in Ayurvedic medicine—has been widely studied and shown to have anti-inflammatory and antioxidant properties.

Consider also the resurgence of interest in the Mediterranean diet, which is rooted in the traditions of Southern Europe. This diet emphasizes whole foods, such as vegetables, fruits, whole grains, and olive oil, alongside moderate fish and dairy consumption. With recent studies linking it to improved heart health and greater longevity, it's clear that there's something profoundly beneficial about the way our ancestors approached food. Today, nutritionists and health experts worldwide advocate these principles, melding historical diet patterns with new scientific research.

As we bridge traditional practices and modern insights, it becomes apparent that many of these remedies address not just the physical dimension of our being but also incorporate elements of mental and emotional well-being. Herbal teas used for relaxation, such as chamomile or lavender, are just as relevant now as they were centuries ago, offering solace amidst today's stressful lifestyles. In this, we find inspiration—not just to reach for the nearest tincture or potion but to understand that true health is holistic, encompassing mind, body, and spirit.

Moreover, the integration of intuitive knowledge with scientific validation is fostering a deeper understanding of why certain practices have endured through millennia. The World Health Organization even recognizes traditional medicine as a part of global health systems, fully aware that these practices may offer affordable and accessible care for many around the world. It's an acknowledgment that the wisdom of the past remains significant and potent even today.

Yet, blending the old with the new does require a fresh perspective. It's about more than blindly following the traditions of yesteryear. It involves a careful examination—utilizing modern methodologies to test and refine these practices to fit today's world. This critical examination is perhaps best exemplified by the increasing acceptance of acupuncture, which, through clinical trials and studies, has gained credibility as an effective treatment for a variety of ailments, from chronic pain to insomnia.

As we continue our journey through natural healing, it's crucial to remember that these remedies are not just alternative solutions but complementary ones. Modern medicine and traditional practices do not have to exist in opposition. Instead, they can work in tandem, offering comprehensive solutions to achieve optimal health. This synergy invites a more balanced and open approach to healing, where each individual's needs and conditions guide the choice of treatment.

The evolution of home remedies from traditional wisdom to modern insights illustrates an enduring truth: our ancestors instinctively understood that healing comes from harmony with the natural world. And while we've achieved extraordinary technological advances, nature remains an unmatched source of healing. By looking to the past, we're not only preserving cultural heritage but also weaving it into the future fabric of wellness and community health.

In embracing this unique intersection of traditional practices and modern insights, we stand to gain not only health and well-being but also a deeper connection with the earth. This legacy invites us to continue exploring, researching, and respecting both the past and present, enhancing our lives with natural, accessible remedies that nurture and sustain.

Chapter 2:
Understanding Herbal Medicine

Delving into the realm of herbal medicine opens doors to a world where nature's bounty becomes an ally in our quest for wellness. Herbal medicine has been woven into the fabric of human healing practices for thousands of years, providing accessible and affordable solutions that align harmoniously with the body's intrinsic balance. It's about understanding how herbs communicate with our bodies to support health and vitality, enhancing our well-being in a gentle yet profound way. As we embrace this journey, we discover that these natural remedies not only address physical ailments but also nurture our mental and emotional health. Exploring key herbs and learning how to grow and harvest our own empowers us to take charge of our health, fostering a deeper connection with the earth. This chapter sets the stage for a transformative embrace of nature's pharmacy, where inspiration and practical knowledge merge to create a blueprint for health that's both sustainable and enriched by tradition.

Key Herbs for Health and Wellness

Harnessing the power of nature, herbal medicine offers an extraordinary path to health and wellness. These gifts from the earth have supported human well-being for centuries, bridging ancient wisdom with modern science. Herbs are more than just plants; they' potent healers that nurture both body and soul. Their potential enhance our lives is vast, and understanding how to integrate th into daily routines can be profoundly empowering.

Let's dive into some key herbs celebrated for their remarkable benefits. First on the list is ginger, renowned for its anti-inflammatory and antioxidant properties. It's a go-to remedy for soothing digestive issues, enhancing circulation, and alleviating nausea. The spicy warmth of ginger doesn't just wake up your senses—it stimulates the body's natural healing processes, making it a versatile addition to any wellness regimen.

Next, we have turmeric, often hailed as the golden spice of life. Turmeric's active compound, curcumin, has been extensively studied for its anti-inflammatory and anti-cancer potential. This bright yellow root is a staple in both culinary arts and natural medicine. Incorporating turmeric into daily meals or as a tea can provide a soothing effect and invigorate the body with its distinctive flavor and healing prowess.

Chamomile is another key herb, famed for its calming effects. Reflecting nature's tender touch, chamomile offers a gentle approach to stress relief and sleep enhancement. Its soothing properties can help ease anxiety and promote relaxation, making it an ideal bedtime ally. A warm cup of chamomile tea invites a comforting ritual, fostering tranquility and restfulness, essential elements of a balanced lifestyle.

Echinacea stands as a symbol of immune support in herbal medicine. Commonly utilized to ward off colds and infections, echinacea is a resilient herb that bolsters the body's defenses. Its use dates back to ancient Indigenous practices, underscoring its enduring relevance in health maintenance. By integrating echinacea into your routine, you arm yourself with a natural shield, fortifying your health against everyday challenges.

In the realm of adaptogens, ashwagandha takes a prominent place. Known for its ability to help the body adapt to stress, ashwagandha promotes balance and vitality. This herb rejuvenates by reducing cortisol levels, enhancing energy, and supporting mental clarity.

Incorporating ashwagandha in supplement form or as a tea can greatly contribute to stress resilience, bringing harmony to mind and body.

Mint, with its refreshing aroma and cooling properties, deserves mention for its digestive benefits. Whether relieving an upset stomach or adding a burst of flavor to dishes and drinks, mint is a versatile herb. Its menthol component induces a soothing sensation, invigorating the senses while aiding digestion. Embracing mint is like inviting a gentle breeze into your wellness practices.

St. John's Wort has gained acclaim for its mood-lifting qualities. As a natural antidepressant, it offers a lifeline to those navigating the depths of sadness or depression. By enhancing neurotransmitter function, St. John's Wort contributes to emotional balance. Its use requires mindfulness of interactions with other medications, but its impact can be transformative for mental health when used appropriately.

Lavender, synonymous with relaxation, not only enchants with its fragrance but also confers therapeutic benefits. Often utilized in aromatherapy, lavender is cherished for its ability to promote calmness and alleviate tension. Its essential oil is widely used in bath salts, lotions, and diffusers, providing a tranquil experience that envelops the senses. Lavender stands as a testament to the healing power of scent.

Beyond these well-known herbs, a lesser spotlighted but equally potent ally is fenugreek. Valued for its ability to lower blood sugar and cholesterol levels, fenugreek seeds are a staple in South Asian cuisine and herbal medicine. Incorporating fenugreek can be as simple as sprinkling the seeds in salads or using them in teas, unlocking a suite of benefits for metabolic health.

Lastly, the magic of garlic should not be underestimated. As a longstanding staple in traditional medicine, garlic is revered for its cardiovascular benefits and antibiotic properties. This robust herb has the power to lower blood pressure, improve cholesterol levels, and support overall cardiac health. Incorporating raw garlic into your diet can amplify its beneficial effects, promoting a heart-healthy lifestyle.

Each of these herbs tells a story: a story of resilience, growth, and the innate wisdom of the earth. By welcoming these natural healers into your life, you're not just complementing conventional medicine but inviting a holistic ethos into your own home. The compassionate practice of herbal medicine not only aids physical healing but inspires a deeper connection to the environment, cultivating gratitude for the earth's bounty.

As you explore the myriad of ways to incorporate these herbs into your routine, remember that wellness is a journey, not a destination. Consider growing your herbs, allowing you to cultivate both health and a deeper understanding of the cycles of nature. Such practices enrich your well-being and provide a sense of fulfillment and self-sufficiency.

In the end, the essence of herbs in health and wellness lies in their ability to harmonize life's rhythms and restore vitality. They're emblematic of a powerful creed: healing with nature's grace. By embracing the subtle and profound changes herbs can usher in, you empower yourself to craft a vibrant tapestry of health that respects and cherishes the world around you.

Growing and Harvesting Your Own Herbs

Growing your own herbs is like opening a door to endless possibilities. Not only does it provide you with fresh ingredients for your remedies, but it also creates a deeper connection with nature and the healing energies of the earth. Imagine stepping out into your garden, inhaling the subtle fragrances, and feeling empowered by knowing that these plants, nurtured by your own hands, will contribute to your health and well-being. It's a practice that marries the ancient wisdom of herbal medicine with modern self-sufficiency.

One of the most satisfying aspects of growing herbs is their versatility. You don't need a sprawling garden to get started. Even a small windowsill can house a thriving herb garden. Begin with hardy herbs like mint, basil, and rosemary, known for their resilience and ability to adapt to indoor environments. As you gain confidence, you can expand your garden to include medicinal herbs like echinacea, lavender, or chamomile, each with unique properties that can enhance your health naturally.

Starting your herb garden requires just a few key steps: choosing the right location, ensuring the right soil conditions, and committing to regular care. Herbs generally thrive in sunny spots with well-drained soil. They favor warmth and light, so pick a location that provides these conditions, or consider using grow lights if you're indoors. As for soil, herbs prefer it slightly alkaline, so you might need to modify your garden's soil by adding lime if necessary. Regular watering and trimming encourage luxurious growth; however, be mindful not to overwater, as most herbs prefer to dry out a bit between waterings.

Once you've planted your herbs, patience is key. Nurturing these plants, watching them sprout and mature, is an exercise in mindfulness. Observe the process; it's reminiscent of life's cycles — organic, rhythmic, and symbiotic. As the days pass, you'll notice each leaf, each stem whispering its readiness to participate in your healing journey. Indeed, this mindful gardening can be as therapeutic as the herbs themselves, offering a refuge from the clamor of daily life.

Harvesting herbs is both an art and a science. Timing is crucial for ensuring the maximum potency of the plant's oils, which embody their therapeutic properties. For most herbs, the best time to harvest is in the morning after the dew has dried but before the sun's heat diminishes the essential oils. Use clean, sharp scissors or pruning shears to avoid damaging the plant. Follow the practice of "taking what you need," ensuring you leave enough of the plant intact to continue growing and regenerating.

Understanding when and how to harvest specific herbs is part of the learning journey. For example, you're encouraged to harvest leafy herbs like basil and mint before they flower, which ensures leaves are tender and flavorful. For flowering herbs like chamomile, pluck the blooms at their peak opening. Remember, preserving harvested herbs properly extends their use and benefits. Drying, freezing, and making tinctures are effective methods to maintain their potency. Hang herbs upside down in a dark, dry place to dry them or use a dehydrator if you prefer a faster method.

Once you've harvested and preserved your herbs, the next step is incorporating them into your daily routine. Fresh or dried, these herbs are versatile players in your health toolkit. Use them to brew healing teas, infuse oils, or create salves and poultices. The simple act of preparing these remedies can deepen your connection with the healing process itself. By crafting your own treatments, you've taken a proactive stance in your journey toward wellness, guided by ancient traditions and your nurtured instincts.

Embracing herbal growth and harvesting rewrites your relationship with medicine. Imagine waking up one morning with a headache and reaching for a sprig of fresh peppermint to relieve your discomfort, or brewing a calming chamomile tea after a particularly stressful day. You have the capability to transform these plants into allies in your quest for a healthier, more balanced life.

Beyond the practical benefits, tending your own herb garden imparts a deeper understanding and appreciation for life's interconnectedness. By growing and harvesting your own herbs, you're participating in a tradition that spans centuries, connecting you to the diverse web of natural healers who came before you. Let this practice encourage curiosity and respect for the natural world, motivating you to explore further into the rich tapestry of herbal knowledge.

In a world increasingly driven by quick fixes, the art of growing and harvesting your own herbs is a gentle reminder of life's simpler yet profound rhythms. It's a meaningful act of self-care, one that fosters independence, nourishes the soul, and elevates health in ways pharmaceuticals often can't replicate. Engage with this practice, savor its rewards, and know that each leaf you nurture brings you closer to a vibrant, empowered existence.

Chapter 3:
Essential Oils and Aromatherapy

As you continue your journey into the world of natural healing, the enchanting realm of essential oils and aromatherapy beckons with its promise of peace and wellness. The age-old practice of using concentrated plant extracts can transform a simple room into a sanctuary of tranquility and health. Essential oils, drawn from nature's most aromatic offerings, provide a multitude of benefits, from calming frazzled nerves to invigorating a weary spirit. Aromatherapy doesn't just cater to the olfactory senses; it influences the mind and body, creating a holistic experience that encourages healing from within. But it's not just about choosing a fragrance—it's about understanding the unique properties each oil possesses and how they can be combined to craft unique, personal blends that cater to your mental and physical needs. This chapter guides you in confidently stepping into this aromatic world, where each essence tells a story, each blend nurtures, and every drop is a step toward a naturally enriched life.

Basics of Essential Oil Use

Essential oils, the aromatic compounds extracted from plants, have the power to transform your environment and well-being in myriad ways. For centuries, these potent liquids have been celebrated for their therapeutic properties, each offering unique benefits that cater to diverse health needs. As part of the art and science of aromatherapy, essential oils invite you to embark on a journey of natural healing, connecting you to the earth's wisdom.

Before you dive into the world of essential oils, it's important to grasp a few key basics that will guide your use. Understanding how to handle these concentrated plant essences ensures that you harness their benefits safely and effectively. With each whirl of scent, you're inviting a balance of mind, body, and spirit.

Let's start by understanding the concept of dilution. Essential oils are incredibly potent, often requiring dilution with a carrier oil like jojoba, coconut, or almond oil before application to the skin. A typical blend might involve several drops of essential oil mixed into a tablespoon of carrier oil. This not only prevents skin irritation but also allows the therapeutic properties of the essential oils to be more slowly and thoroughly absorbed.

Diffusion is another popular method of using essential oils. By dispersing tiny molecules into the air, a diffuser not only fills a room with pleasant aroma but also offers numerous health benefits. Some oils can uplift mood, while others might cleanse the air or support respiratory health. To get started, simply add a few drops of your chosen oil to the diffuser filled with water and let the aroma envelop your space.

Topical application offers direct health benefits to targeted areas of the body. While it requires careful attention to dilution, this method can be particularly effective for soothing sore muscles, easing tension in the head, or promoting skin health. Always conduct a patch test first by applying the diluted oil to a small area of your skin to ensure there is no adverse reaction.

Inhalation is an easy and direct way to experience the immediate impact of essential oils. With just a drop or two on a tissue or a couple of drops in a bowl of steaming water, you can experience their effects through direct inhalation. In moments of stress or congestion, this method offers a quick path to relief.

While exciting, the use of essential oils demands an awareness of safety. Some oils are not recommended for pregnant individuals, children, or those with certain medical conditions. Furthermore, not all oils are safe for internal use. Knowledge and caution serve as your allies in discovering how best to integrate essential oils into your lifestyle.

Storage is another key factor in maintaining the quality and efficacy of your essential oils. Dark glass bottles protect the volatile compounds from sunlight exposure, while a cool, dry environment helps preserve their potency. Properly stored, your essential oils can remain effective for several years.

Engaging with essential oils offers an opportunity for both exploration and mindfulness. By creating a daily or weekly ritual around your use of essential oils, whether it's through a nighttime diffuser blend or a rejuvenating morning face oil, you're actively participating in your own healing journey. This practice not only enhances your physical health but nurtures your emotional and spiritual well-being too.

With endless combinations, the world of essential oils invites exploration. Feel empowered to experiment and discover your own personal blends that resonate with your needs and preferences. As you grow more confident in using these aromatic allies, you may find a favorite synergy of oils that balances your day or a scent that brings tranquility to your evening.

To truly benefit from essential oils, consistent use can play a crucial role. Incorporating them into everyday routines allows you to harness their properties for both acute and preventative care. Whether it involves a warm bath sprinkled with a calming oil or a morning routine accompanied by invigorating scents, the regularity of use enhances their impact over time.

The beauty of essential oils lies not only in their healing potential but also in their ability to inspire a deeper connection with ourselves and nature. As you weave this ancient practice into your modern life, you'll likely discover insights into your own health and well-being, cultivating a sense of harmony and balance that benefits you and those around you.

Essential oils offer more than a momentary escape; they provide tools for nurturing and healing that are grounded in the natural world. So take this knowledge, apply it mindfully, and allow the oils to guide you toward a healthier, more harmonious lifestyle.

Creating Your Own Aromatherapy Blends

Aromatherapy isn't just a science; it's an art that allows you to tap into nature's most fragrant healing powers. When you're delving into the world of essential oils, creating your own blends can be a transformative journey. With each blend, you craft a compact symphony of scents that cater to specific emotional or physical needs. This creative process can be as therapeutic as the blend itself, offering a moment of mindfulness in the midst of life's chaos.

Before you dive into blending, it's crucial to grasp a few fundamental concepts that will guide your creation. Understanding the profiles of oils is paramount. Each essential oil carries with it a history and a quartet of characteristics: aroma, potency, associated health benefits, and personal compatibility. The more you explore these attributes, the more intuitive your blending becomes, allowing you to personalize your own aromatic alchemy.

Start with a purpose. What do you want this blend to achieve? Are you seeking serenity after a long day, invigoration for a morning boost, or perhaps a soothing remedy for tension? Defining your objective will guide your selection of oils. For instance, if you're crafting a sleep blend, lavender, chamomile, and cedarwood might serve your needs.

Begin with a few oils, typically three to five, to keep your blend focused and harmonious. More than five can lead to a muddled mix where individual aromas get lost.

The process of blending is akin to cooking, where the balance of ingredients is key. Use a dropper to add oils drop by drop, and keep a notebook handy to jot down your formulations. Start with a small quantity and adjust as needed. A common approach is the 3-2-1 method: three parts of a base note, two parts of a middle note, and one part of a top note. Base notes, such as vetiver or sandalwood, provide lasting depth. Middle notes like rose or geranium offer warmth and body, while top notes such as lemon or peppermint deliver a fresh first impression.

When blending, pay attention to the intensity of the oils. Some, like peppermint or eucalyptus, are notably strong and should be used sparingly to avoid overpowering your mix. Diluting your essential oils in a neutral carrier oil, such as sweet almond or jojoba, not only helps in dispersing the oils evenly but also ensures safe skin application. A typical dilution is two percent, or about 12 drops of essential oil per ounce of carrier oil for adult use on the skin.

Once you've concocted your blend, allow it to rest for a couple of days to facilitate a full integration of scents. This maturation process is similar to fine wine aging, where time coalesces the aromas into a coherent whole. Afterward, revisit the scent and see if it aligns with your initial vision. Feel free to tweak as necessary; blending is a dynamic exercise that involves a bit of trial and error.

Storage also plays a vital role in maintaining the integrity of your blends. Store them in a cool, dark place, preferably in amber or cobalt blue glass bottles with secured lids. Essential oils are volatile by nature, and light or heat can degrade their efficacy and fragrance over time.

Crafting your own aromatherapy blends is a journey into both the natural world and your senses. While the practice is rooted in simplicity, it paves the way for deep exploration. Each drop you blend is a testament to nature's gifts and your growing intuition. As you hone this skill, not only do you become more attuned to the subtleties of scent and their profound impact on well-being, but you're also empowered with a personalized toolkit for self-care.

Chapter 4:
Healing with Nutrition

In the journey to rejuvenate our bodies and spirits, nutrition stands as a powerful ally. It's fascinating how the bounty of nature can nurture us back to health, sparking vibrant energy where fatigue once lingered. Embracing a diet rich in whole, unprocessed foods, we unlock a treasure trove of healing properties that fortify our immune systems and invigorate our cells. The colors and textures on our plates are not just sustenance but medicine, crafted by earth's wisdom. By choosing the right combinations of nourishing foods, we empower ourselves with the very essence of life. Each meal becomes a ritual of healing and a celebration of vitality, transforming the simple act of eating into a profound experience of self-care and wellness. Let's create a symphony of flavors that harmonizes with our body's innate potential, guiding us gently and effectively toward natural health.

Dietary Principles for Natural Health

In today's fast-paced world, the concept of nourishing the body through natural means serves as a profound, stabilizing force. As we delve deeper into the heart of healing with nutrition, it's essential to embrace dietary principles that not only support physical health but also resonate with our mental and emotional well-being. These principles are grounded in the timeless understanding that food is medicine, a notion that has traversed cultures and centuries, echoing the wisdom of our ancestors. By aligning our diets with nature, we embark on a transformative journey toward holistic health.

At the core of natural dietary practices lies the emphasis on whole foods. Whole foods are those that are unprocessed and unrefined, or processed and refined as little as possible before consumption. These are the foods that retain their nutritional profile and are teeming with life energy. Fruits, vegetables, whole grains, nuts, seeds, and legumes in their closest-to-natural state provide the body with essential vitamins, minerals, fibers, and antioxidants that are crucial for maintaining optimal health. They support the body's natural healing processes, boost immunity, and help ward off chronic diseases.

Balance is another critical principle. It's vital to consume a variety of foods, ensuring that the body gets a wide range of nutrients. By eating a rainbow of colors, different plant foods contribute unique nutritional benefits which collectively enhance vitality. For example, green leafy vegetables are known for their high levels of folate and magnesium, red and orange fruits are rich in antioxidants like vitamin C and beta-carotene, while grains offer heart-protective fibers. This vibrant diversity doesn't just benefit the body; it invigorates the mind and nourishes the soul.

Furthermore, portion control and mindful eating play significant roles in natural health. In a world where supersizing has become the norm, it's essential to reconnect with the body's hunger and fullness cues. Eating mindfully involves taking the time to savor each bite, appreciating the flavors, textures, and aromas, and recognizing the body's signals for hunger and satiety. This practice not only prevents overeating but also fosters a deeper connection with food, transforming meals into moments of gratitude and meditation.

Respecting the natural cycles of the earth can guide us towards seasonally-aligned eating, which is another facet of natural dietary principles. Consuming foods that are in season, and ideally locally sourced, ensures not only the freshness and nutritional quality but also reduces the carbon footprint of our diets. Nature, in its wisdom, provides what we need when we need it the most; consider the bounty of hydration-rich fruits in summer battling heat, or the warmth-invoking root vegetables in the chill of winter.

Incorporating fermented foods is another vital principle. Fermented foods, such as yogurt, sauerkraut, kimchi, and kombucha, are rich in probiotics which support gut health. The gut, often referred to as the second brain, plays a substantial role in overall wellness. Proper gut health aids in digestion, enhances mood, and strengthens the immune system. Embracing these living foods can nurture the microbiome and restore balance within the body.

Another key principle is the reduction of processed sugars and refined grains. These culprits can lead to a host of health issues, including inflammation, weakened immunity, and weight gain. Instead, opt for natural sweeteners like honey or maple syrup in moderation, and choose complex carbohydrates such as whole grains which break down slowly, providing sustained energy and avoiding the spikes and crashes of their refined counterparts.

Hydration should not be overlooked. Water is a fundamental nutrient, vital for every cell, tissue, and organ. It aids in detoxification and supports every function within the body. Encourage the consumption of pure, clean water daily and consider natural herbal teas as a way to stay hydrated while reaping additional health benefits. Herbal teas can calm, invigorate, or even assist in digestion, depending on the herbs chosen.

The principle of balance extends to the nutrients themselves; macronutrients—proteins, fats, and carbohydrates—must be consumed in harmony. Ensuring adequate protein intake, especially from plant sources like beans, legumes, and nuts, supports muscle health and repair. Healthy fats, such as those from avocados, nuts, and seeds, play a critical role in brain health and hormone production. Meanwhile, complex carbohydrates provide the necessary energy for daily activities. This balance is key to sustaining bodily functions and maintaining health.

Incorporating natural dietary principles into daily life requires conscious effort. Begin by gradually introducing these practices rather than overhauling habits overnight, which can be overwhelming. Start with small changes, such as including one extra serving of vegetables at each meal or replacing sugary snacks with fruits or nuts. These incremental adjustments create sustainable habits that ultimately lead to greater health.

It's also beneficial to remember that food is a powerful connector. Sharing a meal with family and friends not only nourishes the body but also nurtures relationships, providing emotional sustenance that is as vital as any other aspect of health. Cooking and eating together encourage the sharing of traditions, laughter, and love, which all enrich the human experience.

The principles outlined here are not about restriction but rather liberation from a state of imbalance. This approach is about rediscovering the joy of eating—celebrating flavors, recognizing the life force in every bite, and finding healing in nature's bounty. It empowers individuals to take charge of their health, aligning body, mind, and spirit in harmony with the natural world.

The journey towards natural health through diet is one of awareness and continuous learning. By embracing these principles, we step into a realm where food is more than just sustenance—it's a vital component of our life's journey, a profound healer, and a testament to the timeless connection between human beings and the earth.

Healing Foods and Their Benefits

When it comes to healing, nature offers an abundance of foods that not only nourish our bodies but also have the power to restore our health. The idea of "food as medicine" isn't new; in fact, it traces back centuries to when our ancestors relied heavily on what the earth provided. Today, we find ourselves rediscovering and, in many ways, rejoicing in these gifts of nature. In this section, we'll explore some of the most remarkable healing foods, their benefits, and how they can be seamlessly integrated into daily life.

First up on our list is garlic, often dubbed nature's antibiotic. With a history as rich as its flavor, garlic packs powerful health benefits thanks to its active compound, allicin. It's known to boost the immune system, which helps in warding off common infections. Research suggests that regular consumption of garlic can help reduce blood pressure and lower cholesterol levels. Incorporating garlic into your meals isn't just about flavor enhancement—it's a step toward better health.

Then there's turmeric, the golden spice that's becoming a staple in many modern diets. It's celebrated for its anti-inflammatory properties, largely due to curcumin, its active ingredient. Curcumin is a natural anti-inflammatory that's as effective as some anti-inflammatory drugs, minus the side effects. Turmeric can be easily added to a variety of dishes, from curries to smoothies, making it a versatile ally in your healing journey.

Balance is key, and nothing exemplifies this better than the humble apple. An apple a day, they say, keeps the doctor away. This saying holds some truth, given that apples are high in fiber and vitamin C while being low in calories. Apples support heart health, promote weight loss, and are linked to a lower risk of diabetes. Whether you enjoy them raw, baked, or juiced, apples are a sweet way to maintain well-being.

Don't forget your greens—leafy vegetables like spinach and kale are nutritional powerhouses. They're packed with vitamins, minerals, and antioxidants. Spinach, known for its high iron content, helps in maintaining healthy blood circulation and strong bones. Kale is rich in vitamins C, A, and K, which are essential for immune function, vision, and bone health, respectively. These greens can be enjoyed in salads, soups, or smoothies for a healthful boost.

Legumes, including beans, lentils, and chickpeas, have been cherished as a protein-rich staple in many cultures. They're high in fiber, which promotes digestive health, and they're a great source of plant-based protein. Consuming legumes regularly can lead to better heart health and decreased risk of chronic diseases. Whether served as a hearty soup or a base for vegetarian dishes, legumes contribute to a balanced diet.

Next, let's dive into the world of berries. Berries such as blueberries, strawberries, and raspberries provide a treasure trove of antioxidants. These fruits contain compounds that combat oxidative stress, reducing the risk of chronic diseases like cancer and heart disease. Berries can be enjoyed fresh, blended into smoothies, or sprinkled over yogurt for an antioxidant-rich treat.

Avocados, with their creamy texture and rich flavor, are more than just tasty—they're packed with monounsaturated fats, which are good for heart health. They help reduce bad cholesterol levels and increase good cholesterol. Moreover, avocados are a great source of potassium, fiber, and vitamins C and K. You can enjoy them in salads, as a toast topping, or directly from their shell with a spoon.

Not to be sidelined, nuts and seeds bring unique health benefits to the table. Almonds, walnuts, chia seeds, and flaxseeds are brimming with healthy fats, protein, and fiber. They're known for supporting heart health, brain function, and managing weight. A small handful as a snack or a sprinkle on your breakfast can make a significant health difference.

Fish, particularly fatty types like salmon, mackerel, and sardines, are superb sources of omega-3 fatty acids, which are crucial for heart and brain health. Regular consumption is associated with a lower risk of heart disease, improved cognitive function, and reduced inflammation. Grilled, baked, or in sushi, fish offers culinary versatility and nutritional value.

Fermented foods like yogurt, kefir, sauerkraut, and kimchi are excellent for gut health. They are rich in probiotics, which foster a healthy balance of gut bacteria. This not only aids digestion but also bolsters the immune system. Incorporating a small serving of fermented foods into your daily diet can be transformative for your gut health.

Don't overlook spices like ginger and cinnamon. Ginger, known for relieving nausea and improving digestion, can also function as an anti-inflammatory aid. Cinnamon helps in reducing blood sugar levels, making it beneficial for those managing diabetes. Adding these spices to tea, desserts, or savory dishes is a simple way to enhance flavor and health.

Finally, let's talk about the role of whole grains such as oats, quinoa, and brown rice. Whole grains are excellent sources of fiber, and they provide essential nutrients like B vitamins and magnesium. They help in maintaining a healthy weight and reducing the risk of heart disease. Including whole grains in your meals ensures sustained energy levels throughout the day.

In conclusion, the beneficial impact of these healing foods stretches beyond simple nutrition. They support various body systems, encourage optimal functioning, and reduce the risk of diseases. The natural bounty we're privileged to access offers a path to healing that is as delicious as it is nourishing. As you embark on this culinary and health journey, remember, integrating these foods into your diet is a gradual process—achieved with intention and perhaps, with a sprinkle of joy.

Chapter 5:
Homeopathic Solutions for
Common Ailments

Navigating the world of homeopathy can feel like unlocking a powerful, well-kept secret where nature's simplicity meets deep wisdom. Imagine having the ability to tap into gentle yet effective remedies right at your fingertips, as you learn to address common ailments with these natural solutions. Whether dealing with a pesky headache or finding relief from seasonal allergies, homeopathy offers a holistic approach that looks beyond symptoms to treat the person as a whole. It empowers you to trust in your body's innate ability to heal with the aid of carefully prepared treatments like arnica for bruises and Chamomilla for teething discomfort. The art of homeopathic healing isn't just about treating the ailment but resonating with natural rhythms and restoring harmony within. As you deepen your understanding and skill in preparing these remedies, you become part of an age-old tradition, embracing an enriched lifestyle where wellness is not about suppressing symptoms but enhancing vitality and balance for a healthy, holistic life.

Key Remedies and Their Applications

Homeopathy is a gentle art that draws upon the subtle energies of nature to restore balance within the body. At its core, it embraces the belief that "like cures like," harnessing highly diluted substances to trigger the body's self-healing ability. The delicate balance between the emotional, physical, and energetic dimensions of our being can often be nudged back into harmony with the right remedy.

One of the most frequently utilized remedies in homeopathy is *Arnica montana*. Known for its remarkable ability to address trauma and bruising, Arnica can truly work wonders. Those who have experienced falls, bumps, or strains might find solace in a carefully administered dose of this remedy. It's not just about healing wounds of the flesh; Arnica ushers a calm to the turmoil beneath, soothing swelling and alleviating the shock that often accompanies physical injuries.

Digestive concerns, a common plight in our fast-paced world, find a friend in *Nux vomica*. This remedy targets ailments associated with overindulgence, whether food, alcohol, or simply the excesses of modern living. Nux vomica assists in easing symptoms such as stomach pain, nausea, and even constipation. Its subtle support guides the stomach and liver back to a state of equilibrium, providing relief and encouraging healthier habits.

When seasonal allergies strike, *Allium cepa*, derived from the humble onion, offers a straightforward solution. Its action mirrors the symptoms it aims to alleviate: watery eyes and a running nose. Just as cutting an onion can bring tears to your eyes, Allium cepa tackles these very symptoms, offering respite from the hay fever that dampens sunny days. Relief is often found with minimal doses, bringing comfort without the side effects sometimes associated with conventional antihistamines.

Cold and flu season prompts an uptick in the use of *Eupatorium perfoliatum*, or boneset. Its name gives a clue to one of its main uses— easing the aching sensation that accompanies severe colds and fevers. Boneset's unique capability to alleviate cruel joint aches and chilling fevers makes it indispensable when you find yourself battling these maladies. Harnessing its soothing nature can lead to faster recovery and a return to vitality.

For those seeking emotional support, *Ignatia amara* shines brightly. Particularly helpful in managing the aftermath of grief, worry, or disappointment, Ignatia helps mend the spirit by alleviating associated symptoms like headaches, throat tightness, and even erratic mood swings. This remedy encourages a journey towards emotional resilience, offering solace during times of heartache and distress.

Travelers often turn to *Cocculus indicus* for relief from motion sickness. Whether by air, sea, or land, the unpleasant dizziness and nausea that can accompany long journeys melt away with Cocculus. This remedy not only abates symptoms in the short-term, aiding travelers to enjoy their adventures but also presents a path to long-term adjustment to motion.

Insomnia and restless nights find an adversary in *Coffea cruda*. Derived from the coffee bean, Coffea counters the very stimulations one might expect from caffeine. In small amounts, it works to calm an overactive mind, enabling a peaceful transition into sleep. The busy mind, once quietened, allows the body to relax, aiding in the sacred renewal of rest.

For skin irritations, *Calendula officinalis*, also known as the marigold, reveals its worth through its calming properties. It possesses natural antiseptic and anti-inflammatory traits, promoting the healing of cuts, burns, and other skin afflictions. Calendula can even be used topically to utilize its soothing efficacy further, mending the skin while restoring its vitality.

Aconitum napellus becomes crucial when combating sudden onset fevers or the early stages of a cold, especially those brought on by exposure to cold wind. The classic situation where Aconite proves its supremacy is when symptoms arise suddenly and with great intensity, accompanied by restlessness and anxiety. Quelling these early signs can often prevent more serious illnesses from taking hold.

Chamomilla provides relief for teething infants or irritable adults. Its calming influence helps in matters of oversensitivity, particularly when physical pain is accompanied by irritability, anger, or impatience. Soothe the storm within by administering Chamomilla precisely when frustration turns into an emotional tempest.

Rhus toxicodendron, made from poison ivy, paradoxically offers relief for arthritis pain and stiffness. Those who experience significant discomfort upon initially moving but feel relief once they get going often find Rhus tox a dependable ally. This powerful remedy helps shake off the morning sluggishness, easing into a rhythm of more comfortable, fluid mobility.

Finally, when your life feels like it's spinning out of grasp, *Gelsemium sempervirens* can steady the ship. A remedy for the fearful, those anticipating challenging events, or individuals facing the unknown with nervous anticipation, Gelsemium fortifies courage. It's a gentle coaxing into calmness, urging a serene and steady approach to the tasks ahead.

These remedies exemplify the heart of homeopathy—each harnessing the vibrant energies of nature towards healing and balance. They remind us that modern life's ailments often have ancient solutions waiting patiently for us to rediscover them. Embrace these remedies as allies on your journey toward brighter health, knowing they serve not only to amend singular symptoms but to promote genuine wellness on every level.

Preparing Homeopathic Treatments

Homeopathy has been capturing the interest of many who seek to bolster their health with the gentle power of nature. At its core, homeopathy is an art and science, blending precise ingredients and potencies to align with the body's inherent healing abilities. As we navigate the world seeking harmony and well-being, preparing homeopathic treatments in your own home can be both a rewarding and empowering journey.

The first step in preparing homeopathic treatments is understanding the principles of homeopathic dilution and potentization. Unlike conventional medicine, where more active ingredients are believed to correlate with stronger effects, homeopathy trusts in the opposite. The principle of "like cures like" postulates that a substance causing symptoms in a healthy person could, when highly diluted, treat similar symptoms in a sick person. This involves diluting a substance in water or alcohol and then vigorously shaking it, a process known as succussion. The belief is that, through dilution, the essence of the substance is magnified while its potential toxicity is minimized, rendering what some describe as energy or vibrational medicine.

When you're ready to start concocting your own remedies, finding the right ingredients is key. Most homeopathic substances are derived from natural sources: plants, minerals, and animals. These ingredients, known as mother tinctures, are quite potent in their unprocessed state. Thus, they must be handled with care and respect, acknowledging their potent potential to affect the body's delicate balance.

Next, the selection of potencies in homeopathic treatments requires discerning consideration. Homeopathic remedies are available in varying potencies, expressed as ratios like 6C, 12C, 30C, and even 200C. Lower potencies are generally suited for physical symptoms and more frequent administration, whereas higher potencies typically address emotional or chronic conditions with less frequent dosage. Choosing the correct potency is a finely-tuned process that considers the nature of the ailment as well as the individual's overall energy.

It's also essential to have the proper tools and materials on hand for home remedy preparation. This includes clean glass bottles for storage, pure ethanol or distilled water for dilutions, and high-quality homeopathic blanks or sugar pellets for dosing. These sugar pellets are typically impregnated with the potentized liquid remedy. Organization and meticulousness during preparation ensure both the purity and efficacy of the remedy, as anything less might compromise the intended benefits.

Storing your homeopathic remedies correctly is just as crucial as their initial preparation. Remedies should be kept in a cool, dark place away from direct sunlight and strong odors. Proper storage not only preserves their effectiveness but also ensures they are safe and ready to use when needed. Homeopathic remedies, due to their unique nature, retain their potency for a long duration when stored under optimal conditions, offering years of homeopathic support.

Moreover, understanding the timing and dosage in administering homeopathic remedies can significantly influence results. While homeopathy generally advocates for lower doses over prolonged periods, the frequency of dosage might change depending on the severity of the symptoms. Acute conditions might demand a more frequent dosage until signs start subsiding, while chronic ailments might involve less regular administration over a longer time frame. Trusting in the body's intimate connection with its own needs, guided by careful observation and adjustment, enhances the efficacy of any homeopathic treatment.

Combining remedies, when necessary, is another aspect to consider. Although traditional homeopathy often relies on single remedies, some modern approaches advocate the use of combinations to address complex presentations. This approach requires a nuanced understanding of how different remedies can synergize or, conversely, counteract each other. Always ensure that any combination does not dilute the specific action of each remedy. If in doubt, consultation with a seasoned homeopath could offer valuable insights into this delicate art.

Lastly, it's important to approach this practice with mindfulness and intention. Preparing and administering homeopathic remedies involves more than just physical actions; it is a holistic practice that engages both the heart and mind. Recognize the interconnectedness of the physical, emotional, and spiritual dimensions in homeopathy. As you delve deeper into preparing homeopathic treatments, cultivate an attitude of reflection and patience. These qualities, combined with knowledge and care, can transform the way you perceive health and healing.

Incorporating homeopathy into your life offers a journey that's both personal and profound. It provides the tools to explore natural paths towards health and rejuvenation, enhancing your capacity to live harmoniously with the world around you. Whether you're addressing a simple cold or nurturing long-term well-being, preparing homeopathic treatments is a testament to the body's remarkable ability to heal and the nurturing power found in nature's embrace.

Chapter 6:
The Role of Supplements in Wellness

Supplements have quietly woven themselves into the fabric of modern wellness, offering a bridge between our daily diets and the nutrients our bodies crave for optimal health. While whole foods remain the cornerstone of a natural approach to healing, the judicious use of supplements can provide targeted support, enhancing vitality and resilience. In understanding their role, it's vital to recognize that not all supplements are created equal. The journey to wellness involves selecting high-quality, natural options that align with individual health needs and goals. Armed with the right information, supplements can complement a holistic lifestyle, empowering you to take proactive steps in nurturing your well-being and reducing reliance on pharmaceuticals. Striking a thoughtful balance between traditional wisdom and modern science, supplements become more than just quick fixes; they transform into purposeful allies on the path to long-lasting health and tranquility.

Understanding Supplements for Health

In the intricate tapestry of natural healing, supplements have emerged as vital threads, weaving together centuries-old practices with modern wellness insights. Supplements, in their myriad forms, have become treasured allies in the quest for health and vitality. While they can't replace whole foods, they serve to fortify diets, fill nutritional gaps, and aid in the prevention and management of various health conditions.

Understanding the role and efficacy of supplements is essential for anyone eager to embrace a balanced approach to health.

One of the cornerstones of comprehending supplements is acknowledging the diversity they offer. They range from simple vitamins and minerals to more complex compounds like probiotics and herbal extracts. Vitamins, such as vitamin C or the B-complex group, often top the list for their direct impact on bodily functions. Minerals like magnesium and zinc are critical for countless biochemical processes that sustain life. Meanwhile, herbal supplements reintroduce us to the plants our ancestors relied upon for healing.

The importance of supplements lies not just in what they provide but also in how they interact with the body. For instance, antioxidants are powerful in protecting cells against damage from free radicals. These free radicals are unstable molecules that can lead to chronic diseases if left unchecked. By consuming antioxidant-rich supplements, individuals can stave off oxidative stress, fostering an internal environment conducive to health and longevity.

Nonetheless, supplements do more than just bridge nutritional gaps. They empower individuals to take proactive steps in managing their health. For instance, omega-3 fatty acids, commonly found in fish oil supplements, are renowned for supporting cardiovascular health. In our fast-paced world, where stress abounds and fatty diets are common, these supplements offer an invaluable defense against heart disease.

Yet, as you dive deeper into the world of supplements, it's crucial to maintain a discerning eye. The supplement market is vast, with countless options claiming miraculous results. Critical thinking is your compass. Not all supplements are created equal, and research-backed products should always take precedence over unsubstantiated claims. Always opt for supplements that have been rigorously tested and certified by regulatory bodies. This ensures safety and efficacy.

Understanding how supplements interact with your unique body composition can transform your health journey. Everyone's biochemical makeup is different, meaning that what works well for one person might not yield the same results for another. A key aspect of this involves consulting with healthcare practitioners who understand these intricacies. They can offer insights tailored to your needs, helping you choose supplements that align with your health goals.

Moreover, timing often plays a vital role in supplement efficacy. Some supplements are best absorbed when taken with food, while others require an empty stomach for optimal absorption. Calcium, for example, is best taken in smaller doses throughout the day rather than in one large dose. Understanding these nuances empowers you to maximize the benefits derived from each supplement.

Integrity and mindfulness in dosage are equally critical. While the allure of quick fixes can be tempting, it's important to remember that more isn't always better. Over-supplementation can lead to toxicity and cause adverse effects, negating the benefits you seek. It's about balance, logic, and a keen insight into your body's requirements.

As we explore the realm of supplements, it's equally inspiring to realize the way they complement other natural practices. Integrative health involves harmonizing supplements with nutrition, exercise, and mental well-being. For instance, working in tandem with meditation and yoga, adaptogenic herbs like Ashwagandha can help reduce stress and improve resilience, creating a symphony of healing that elevates both body and mind.

Furthermore, access to supplements isn't exclusive to synthetic forms. You can look to nature by cultivating herbs like Echinacea or Turmeric in your own backyard. This not only ensures the purity of what you ingest but also deepens your understanding of the natural world. By doing so, you engage with nature's pharmacy directly, harnessing its bounty for personalized health solutions.

As we continue to explore the depths of supplements for health, let us not overlook the importance of mindful consumerism and sustainability. Ethical harvesting and sourcing practices ensure that the benefits of these supplements do not come at the expense of the environment or local communities. Supporting brands that prioritize fair-trade and eco-friendly practices fosters a healthier planet alongside personal health.

Integrating supplements into your life isn't about chasing every new trend. Rather, it's about coming into a harmonious relationship with your own body and its needs. It's about listening, understanding, and responding thoughtfully to what will truly enhance your well-being. Through this enlightened approach, you not only bolster your health today but lay the foundation for a future where natural wisdom guides every step of your wellness journey.

In this evolving dialogue with nature, the journey of understanding supplements becomes an exploration of possibility. To embrace supplements is to take a courageous step into a world of vibrant health, leveraging the old wisdom while welcoming the new. It's an inspiring interplay of knowledge, compassion, and self-discovery, where each choice reverberates with the potential to nurture life's greatest gift—our health.

Choosing Quality Natural Supplements

Selecting the right natural supplements is an empowering journey that enhances our wellness ambitions. It's not just about adding pills or powders to your daily routine, but about choosing products that align with a holistic view of health. In a world overflowing with supplement options, the quest for quality is crucial.

The first step in this journey is understanding what you truly need. Our bodies are unique ecosystems, and recognizing your specific health requirements can direct you toward the appropriate supplements. For example, someone with a vitamin D deficiency might prioritize this supplement over an array of herbal blends. Personalization is key.

Once you've pinpointed your needs, sourcing quality products becomes paramount. With countless brands on the market, it's essential to read labels meticulously. Look for supplements that list active ingredients clearly and avoid those with fillers and artificial additives. Transparency in labeling usually indicates a reputable product. Respect the journey of your supplement from raw material to bottle; brands with ethical sourcing often indicate quality conscience.

Third-party testing seals are another beacon of assurance. Certifications from organizations such as NSF International or ConsumerLab confirm that the supplement underwent rigorous testing for purity and potency. These seals ensure that what's on the label matches what's in the bottle. It's akin to having an honest friend vouch for your choice.

Consider how natural processing methods impact supplement quality. Cold-pressed oils and non-GMO sources maintain the efficacy of vitamins and minerals better than their highly processed counterparts. Natural extraction methods preserve the integrity of herbs, ensuring that they retain their healing properties.

In your selection process, remember the synergy of supplements. Some nutrients require companions to fully benefit the body. For instance, calcium needs vitamin D for optimal absorption. Understanding these relationships can make your supplementation more effective and holistic, further enhancing your wellness journey.

Dosage is another factor that can't be overstated. It's tempting to think that more of a good thing is better, but this mindset can be counterproductive, even dangerous. Tailor your dosage to your body's specific requirements, which can be influenced by factors like age, activity level, and existing health conditions. Knowledgeable healthcare practitioners play an invaluable role in determining the right dosage.

Before diving into the supplement industry's vast offerings, seek guidance from a trusted healthcare professional. A healthcare expert familiar with your individual health picture can suggest necessary supplements while avoiding those that might interact negatively with existing conditions or medications.

As we delve deeper into the world of quality natural supplements, it's vital to approach it with both curiosity and caution. The relationship you build with supplements can be a powerful partnership in your journey toward wellness. Let your choices reflect not only current health needs but also your broader wellness vision.

Engaging with natural supplements should not feel like a chore, but rather like nurturing a dialogue between nature and living tissue. It's an invitation to explore the bounty of the earth while respecting our body's wisdom.

Furthermore, staying informed about the latest research and developments in natural supplements can greatly benefit your decisions. The field evolves rapidly, with new findings challenging old assumptions and leading to more effective, safer supplements. Subscribe to reputable wellness publications and community forums to ensure you're always updated.

If faced with skepticism or doubts, remember that this journey is deeply personal. What's profound is recognizing that every step toward a natural supplement routine is a stride towards self-awareness and harmony with nature. Embrace this odyssey with an open yet discerning mind, guided by both science and instinct.

In the end, choosing quality natural supplements is about aligning your choices with your health goals and values. It's about enhancing your body's natural healing power with mindful support. Let these choices speak to a commitment to wellness that appreciates the delicate balance of nature and our own inherent capacity to maintain health.

The landscape of natural supplements is as much about personal growth as it is about health. As you embrace these choices, you become akin to a gardener, nurturing and cultivating your own well-being with every informed, careful decision. May your path be both instructive and nourishing, leading you toward a harmonious and vibrant life.

Chapter 7:
Mind-Body Connection in
Natural Healing

The interplay between mind and body forms the essence of natural healing, encouraging a harmonious relationship that fosters complete well-being. Understanding this connection empowers individuals to not only heal but thrive, by tapping into the synergy of mental clarity and physical vitality. Techniques such as mindfulness and meditation serve as powerful tools, helping bridge the gap between mental states and physical health. When practiced consistently, these methods bolster resilience, reduce stress, and cultivate inner peace, setting the stage for natural healing to occur. By embracing this connection, you can unlock an intrinsic ability to nurture and restore holistic health, reinforcing the idea that wellness truly begins within. This mind-body integration is not just a concept but a practical strategy that can transform and invigorate every aspect of life.

Techniques for Mental and Physical Well-being

Exploring the mind-body connection reveals how intricately linked our mental and physical states are. This interdependence forms the backbone of natural healing, advocating for holistic approaches that respect the unity of body and mind. Techniques for nurturing both mental and physical well-being are as varied as they are invaluable, offering pathways to enhance health through natural and mindful living.

One profound technique that stands out is the practice of *breathwork*. The simple act of paying attention to one's breath can wield transformative power. Slow, intentional breathing calms the mind and reduces stress, while also lowering blood pressure and improving circulation. By practicing rhythmic breathing each day, individuals can harness a tool that's both readily accessible and incredibly effective.

In addition to breathwork, physical movement plays a crucial role in aligning the mind and body. **Yoga and Tai Chi**, ancient practices celebrated for promoting balance, flexibility, and tranquility, offer more than just physical benefits. They engage the mind, encouraging a meditative state that fosters greater self-awareness and mental clarity. Through consistent practice, these movements cultivate a holistic sense of peace and well-being, demonstrating the profound healing potential found in the marriage of mind and body.

The gentle art of self-compassion is another pillar of mental wellness. Encouraging kindness towards oneself reduces feelings of anxiety and depression and can significantly enhance overall life satisfaction. Embracing imperfection and treating oneself with the same compassion extended to a friend can lead to profound mental healing. When coupled with other techniques, self-compassion reinforces resilience and positive self-regard.

An often overlooked yet powerful technique is *journaling*. This simple habit provides an outlet for emotions, helping individuals process thoughts and experiences that might otherwise weigh heavily on the mind. By externalizing worries onto paper, there is a cathartic release that can promote mental clarity and peace. Journaling can also aid in identifying patterns and triggers, allowing for deeper self-reflection and personal growth.

For those seeking to build a strong mental and physical foundation, **nature therapy** offers an enticing option. Immersing oneself in natural environments has been shown to reduce stress and anxiety, while simultaneously boosting mood and cognitive function. The tranquility of nature instills a sense of calm that's hard to replicate in urban settings. Whether it's a walk in the park or a hike through the woods, communing with nature can lead to rejuvenation and healing.

Mindfulness and meditation deserve special mention for their profound impact on mental and physical health. Meditative practices lead to a heightened state of awareness and a reduction in negative thoughts. Simple routines, such as focused breathing or visualization, allow individuals to center themselves, fostering a sense of calm that permeates through both mind and body. The benefits of meditation are far-reaching, including improved focus, better emotional health, and even enhanced pain management.

Nourishing the body with the right *nutrition* is another technique that cannot be overlooked. A balanced diet rich in fruits, vegetables, and whole grains provides the body with essential nutrients that support not just physical health but mental well-being as well. Omega-3 fatty acids, for example, have been linked to reduced symptoms of depression, while antioxidants from fruits and vegetables help combat stress. Eating mindfully, being present with each bite, further connects the act of nourishment with appreciation and gratitude.

Acupuncture, a cornerstone of traditional Chinese medicine, also outlines the inseparable link between mind and body. By stimulating specific points on the body, acupuncture promotes the flow of energy or "Qi," leading to improved emotional balance and physical health. Many find this practice helpful for relieving pain, promoting relaxation, and enhancing overall wellness.

Let's not forget the importance of quality *sleep*. Sleep is the body's natural healer, playing a critical role in emotional regulation and physical recovery. Developing good sleep hygiene—like maintaining a regular sleep schedule, creating a restful environment, and avoiding screens before bedtime—can drastically improve one's health. Quality sleep restores energy, sharpens concentration, and elevates mood, forming a crucial pillar of well-being.

In conclusion, weaving these techniques into daily life may offer profound benefits that extend far beyond immediate gratification. Each method, from simple breathwork to more involved practices like yoga, contributes to a more balanced state of being. Together, they cultivate a harmonious connection between mind and body, empowering individuals to take charge of their health in an enriching, natural way. With commitment and mindfulness, the journey towards enhancing mental and physical well-being becomes not just a goal but a fulfilling process of self-discovery and healing.

Incorporating Mindfulness and Meditation

In an age where the pace of life seems to quicken with each passing day, the practice of mindfulness and meditation serves as an oasis—a brief yet profound pause to reconnect with oneself. It's a bridge between the mind and body that facilitates natural healing, advocating for presence in every moment. But what exactly is mindfulness, and why is it so pivotal in the realm of natural healing?

Mindfulness is the practice of purposefully paying attention to the present moment without judgment. It's about tuning into here and now, acknowledging thoughts and feelings as transient experiences rather than permanent states. This practice allows individuals to break free from the cycle of constant rumination, which can lead to stress and anxiety, and instead cultivate a sense of peace and clarity.

Meditation, often intertwined with mindfulness, is an ancient practice that dates back thousands of years. It's a method to train the mind, seeking to alter our habitual patterns of thinking and perception. Meditation comes in many forms, such as guided sessions, focused breathing, or even visualization, each offering unique ways to clear the mental clutter and foster inner tranquility.

Evidence of meditation's benefits is not just anecdotal; there is a growing body of research supporting its role in health and healing. Regular meditation has been shown to reduce the symptoms of anxiety and depression, enhance concentration, and even improve physical health by lowering blood pressure and boosting the immune system. It's a holistic tool that nurtures both mind and body.

A simple way to incorporate mindfulness into daily life is through breathing exercises. Begin by finding a comfortable seat and closing your eyes. Breathe deeply, in through the nose and out through the mouth. Focus on the sensation of each breath—the rise and fall of your chest. If your mind starts to wander, gently bring your attention back to your breathing. Even just a few minutes a day can make a significant difference.

Mindfulness can also be embedded in daily activities. Consider mindful walking: focus on each step, the feel of the ground beneath your feet, the rhythm of your movement. This intentional awareness transforms a simple walk into a meditation, gifting moments of peace and presence regardless of where you are or how busy your schedule may be.

The beautiful thing about meditation is that it's highly adaptable. It doesn't require a special time or place. Some find peace in guided meditations offered in apps or online, while others prefer tranquil moments enveloped by nature. The key is consistency—regular practice yields the most profound benefits.

For those new to mindfulness, creating a dedicated space for practice can be beneficial. Choose a quiet, comfortable corner of your home and minimize distractions. Decorate with calming elements— perhaps a soft cushion, a gentle candle, or a soothing fragrance from essential oils. This space becomes a sanctuary, a place to retreat and recharge.

Mindfulness and meditation are particularly powerful in reducing stress—one of the most significant barriers to healing. When stress is chronic, our bodies remain in a heightened state of alert, inhibiting the body's natural ability to repair and heal. By calming the mind through these practices, we foster an internal environment where healing can occur naturally and effectively.

For those who struggle with consistent practice, starting with short, manageable sessions is advised. As little as five minutes of focused meditation can begin to shift your mindset and improve well-being. Over time, these moments become more natural, and the duration can be gradually increased.

Sharing meditation practices with others can enhance its effects. Group meditation or mindfulness sessions create a shared energy and sense of community. Whether with family, friends, or a local group, practicing together can deepen connections and enhance your commitment to personal well-being.

Incorporating mindfulness and meditation into one's lifestyle is more than just a remedy—it's a preventative strategy. It guards against the emotional toll of life's challenges and maintains a harmonious balance between mind and body. It's about transforming daily habits into opportunities for intentional living.

The journey to incorporating mindfulness and meditation doesn't end with understanding or even daily practice. It's an evolving path that constantly invites deeper exploration and refinement. As you grow with your practice, it becomes entwined with your very approach to life, influencing how you interact with the world, others, and yourself.

As you explore this dimension of healing, remember that the goal isn't perfection but presence. Embrace each step of your mindfulness journey and recognize that every moment spent in presence is a step towards holistic health. The mind-body connection in natural healing is framed by moments like these—simple, powerful, and transformative.

Chapter 8:
Natural Remedies for Skin Care

In the gentle art of nurturing your skin, nature offers profound gifts that embrace simplicity and efficacy. Just as a painter strokes a canvas with care, you too can apply natural remedies that transform your skin into a vibrant masterpiece. Harnessing the power of ingredients from your kitchen or garden, like soothing aloe vera or invigorating mint, brings not only radiance but also a sense of empowerment. These remedies, rooted in both tradition and science, offer solutions for common issues like dryness or blemishes. By choosing natural alternatives, you're reducing reliance on synthetic products, which can often harbor hidden irritants. Instead, embrace the beauty that comes from within, encouraged by the timeless wisdom that healing and harmony with nature needn't be a journey of complexity. Let your skin be a testament to the love and care you've given yourself, woven with nature's own enduring touch.

Homemade Skin Treatments and Tips

Our skin, an inexhaustible communication channel between our bodies and the environment, requires attentive care. It tells stories, letting us know when we're stressed, ill, or in need of a little TLC. With numerous skincare products on the market, it can be overwhelming to choose wisely. Fortunately, nature offers a treasure trove of ingredients that nurture our skin gently and effortlessly. This section delves into homemade treatments, rich with vitamins, minerals, and natural compounds, to help enhance your skin's health and vitality.

Let's begin with the versatile wonders of honey. Honey isn't just for sweetening your tea; it's a potent natural humectant, meaning it locks in moisture, keeping your skin hydrated and soft. Known for its antibacterial properties, a honey mask can help reduce inflammation and clear minor breakouts. Simply apply a thin layer of raw honey to your face, let it sit for about 15 minutes, and rinse with warm water. You'll likely find your skin feeling smoother, plumped, and refreshed.

Another cornerstone of natural skincare is the humble aloe vera plant. Often lauded for its healing properties, aloe vera gel can be used directly from the leaf as an effective treatment for sunburns, minor cuts, or as a daily moisturizer. Its soothing, cooling effect makes it a wonderful choice, especially for sensitive or irritated skin. For a simple, soothing facial mask, mix a tablespoon of aloe vera gel with a teaspoon of honey. This combination not only calms the skin but also enhances its natural glow.

Delving into the kitchen pantry, you'll find oats, an often-overlooked miracle worker for your skin. Ground oats make an excellent base for DIY facial scrubs and masks, bringing gentle exfoliation and soothing relief to irritated skin. To create a calming oatmeal mask, blend 1/3 cup of oats into a fine powder and mix with half a cup of hot water. Once it cools, add a tablespoon of plain yogurt and a tablespoon of honey. Apply the mixture evenly to your face, leaving it for about 10 minutes before rinsing. Your skin should feel calm, clean, and nourished.

Arguably, one of the most exciting parts of natural skincare is the endless combinations and customizations you can explore to suit your skin's unique needs. Essential oils such as tea tree, lavender, and chamomile frequently play roles in these custom solutions. Tea tree oil, with its antimicrobial properties, blends well with a coconut oil base to tackle acne. A couple of drops of lavender oil in a carrier oil like jojoba or almond can promote relaxation and reduce redness. Chamomile oil, celebrated for its calming attributes, works wonders for sensitive skin when added to a homemade moisturizer.

Fruit enzymes also hold powerful properties that can transform your skincare routine. Take papaya, for instance, which contains the enzyme papain, known for its ability to gently exfoliate, removing dead skin cells and brightening skin tone. To concoct a simple papaya mask, mash a small piece of ripe papaya and apply it to the skin for 5-10 minutes. Rinse it off with lukewarm water to reveal a radiant complexion.

Although often underrated, understanding the role of proper hydration and dietary influences is pivotal for maintaining healthy skin. Drinking adequate water throughout the day ensures that your skin stays hydrated from the inside out. Coupled with a balanced diet rich in omega-3 fatty acids, antioxidants, vitamins, and minerals, these elements lay the groundwork for a luminous, healthy complexion. A diet abundant in fruits, vegetables, nuts, and seeds significantly supports skin health, arguably more than any topical treatment alone.

Beyond physical treatments, fostering a harmonious mind-body connection—the intersection where mental wellness contributes to physical appearance—enhances overall skin health. Practices such as mindfulness meditation can manage stress levels, reducing the production of stress hormones that can compromise skin integrity. Regular practice of stress-reducing techniques is a subtle yet profound complement to your skincare regimen, embodying a holistic approach to wellness that radiates beauty from within.

As you explore these homemade treatments and tips, remember the uniqueness of your skin. What suits one person may not suit another, and part of the beauty of natural remedies is the ability to tailor treatments to meet your specific needs. Be patient and allow time for your skin to respond to these natural ingredients. You're not just experimenting with skincare solutions; you're embarking on a transformative journey to reconnect with the earth's abundant offerings.

In a world where skincare can often be costly and bewildering, stepping back to embrace homemade treatments is empowering. With just a few simple ingredients, a dash of creativity, and a commitment to nurturing your skin naturally, you can achieve a healthier, more vibrant complexion. So, delve into your pantry, garden, or local market, and start your journey of natural skincare tailored just for you. Your skin will speak volumes of gratitude.

Herbal Solutions for Common Skin Issues

When it comes to caring for the largest organ of our body—our skin— nature offers an array of incredible solutions. Herbs have been revered for centuries for their potent healing properties. They provide a gentle, yet effective approach to tackling various skin issues, many of which are common and often frustrating. Rashes, acne, eczema, and even minor burns can benefit from the soothing touch of botanicals, acting not only as remedies but also as daily enhancements to our skin routine.

Let's start with everyone's favorite: **aloe vera**. The gel from this succulent plant has been nicknamed "the burn plant" for a reason. It's naturally soothing and healing, perfect for sunburns or any heat-related skin irritation. Simply apply the fresh gel from a broken leaf directly onto the affected area. It cools, hydrates, and works almost instantaneously to reduce inflammation. This wonder herb should be a staple in every home's natural medicine cabinet.

Another common issue is acne, a condition that doesn't discriminate and affects individuals across age groups. Here, nature steps in with **tea tree oil**. Derived from the leaves of the Melaleuca plant, tea tree oil boasts impressive antiseptic properties. A dab of this oil on blemishes can help detoxify pores and reduce outbreaks. Mixing a drop with a carrier oil can enhance its effectiveness while preventing potential skin irritation due to its concentrated potency.

Calendula is another herb that deserves a moment in the spotlight, especially for those dealing with dry or inflamed skin. Known for its vibrant orange flowers, calendula is rich in flavonoids, contributing to its anti-inflammatory and hydration-boosting capabilities. A calendula-infused cream or lotion can help alleviate the itchiness associated with eczema and encourage overall skin health. Regular application can create a protective barrier on the skin, allowing it to retain moisture and recover at its natural pace.

For those battling more persistent skin conditions like psoriasis, **chamomile** can be a source of immense relief. This gentle herb, often synonymous with relaxation, also offers powerful anti-inflammatory and antimicrobial properties. A chamomile-infused oil can be applied to affected areas to calm redness and scaling, allowing the skin to heal more comfortably. Its calming effect is not just limited to the skin; inhaling the aroma can help alleviate stress, which often exacerbates skin conditions.

Herbal solutions are not limited to external applications. Internal health reflects on the skin too, so incorporating herbs like **burdock root** can enhance your natural skincare regimen from the inside out. Burdock root acts as a blood purifier, helping to cleanse toxins that can manifest as skin issues. Adding burdock root to teas or tinctures can support overall skin health and manifest clearer, more radiant skin.

Prepared to try a DIY remedy at home? Consider concocting a **witch hazel**-based toner. Witch hazel is an astringent praised for its ability to tighten pores and reduce oil production. A homemade toner with witch hazel, infused with herbs like lavender or rose petals, offers a refreshing, balancing concoction that can be used daily to maintain skin clarity and elasticity.

Even minor cuts and bruises can become focal points for herbal healing. **Comfrey**, often referred to as "knitbone," is an unparalleled healer thanks to allantoin, which supports the growth of new skin cells. Comfrey's leaves can be crushed to create a poultice or infused into an ointment to promote rapid healing of cuts, scrapes, and bruises.

In instances where hyperpigmentation or uneven skin tone becomes a concern, **turmeric** arrives as a vibrant solution. Its active component, curcumin, has been studied for its ability to lighten dark spots and provide an overall luminous glow. A simple homemade mask combining yogurt and turmeric can help brighten and even out skin tone over time. It's a radiant elixir straight from nature's bounty.

Cucumber, often overlooked as an herb, is a fantastic addition too, known for its hydration and cooling properties. It provides instant relief for puffy eyes and tired skin. Preparing a simple paste of cucumber juice mixed with herbal teas can serve as an excellent face mask to rejuvenate and refresh glowing skin after a long day.

The journey to transforming skin through these herbal solutions isn't just a shift from conventional methods; it's a reconnection with Earth's innate wisdom. Each herb carries a signature gift, and when used thoughtfully, these gifts illuminate both the skin and the spirit.

Seeking plant-based alternatives allows us to not only treat common skin concerns but also invites a holistic approach to beauty and wellness. It empowers us to believe in the nurturing power of nature, inspiring hope in what our ancestors knew all along—herbs, with their simple elegance and profound effectiveness, have the answers.

Chapter 9:
Household Remedies for
Everyday Health

In the gentle embrace of nature, we find an abundance of household remedies that nurture our daily well-being. Imagine your home transformed into a sanctuary of health, where simple, yet profound, solutions offer respite from everyday ailments. From the soothing comfort of a warm ginger tea to ease a troubled stomach, to a whiff of eucalyptus that clears the mind and air, these remedies are accessible treasures. Crafting a natural medicine cabinet becomes an act of empowerment, where you curate not just items but a lifestyle that honors simplicity and efficacy. Each remedy chosen echoes ancestral wisdom, yet fits seamlessly into modern living, addressing common concerns with a caring touch. By embracing these natural allies, you embark on a journey that inspires confidence and vitality, proving that within the ordinary lies extraordinary potential for health.

Creating a Natural Medicine Cabinet

Imagine opening your medicine cabinet and seeing a bounty of natural remedies available at your fingertips, each a testament to the power of nature. Transitioning from synthetic pharmaceuticals to natural solutions doesn't just offer a healthier approach; it supports a more sustainable lifestyle too. Creating a natural medicine cabinet isn't just about replacing one remedy with another. It's about understanding the holistic harmony each ingredient brings and how it can contribute to your overall well-being.

Stocking up on essential oils can be a great start. Lavender oil, for instance, works wonders for soothing minor burns, while peppermint oil can relieve headaches and digestive discomfort. These oils are versatile and potent, making them invaluable tools in any natural medicine cabinet. But remember, quality matters. Choose organic, therapeutic-grade oils where possible; they ensure purity and potency, offering the most therapeutic benefits.

Herbal tinctures are another cornerstone of a natural medicine cabinet. Made by soaking herbs in alcohol or vinegar, these liquid extracts capture the essence of the plant's healing power. Tinctures are easy to administer, with a long shelf life, and they can work wonders for a variety of ailments. Echinacea tincture, for example, is excellent for boosting the immune system during cold and flu season, while valerian root can help promote restful sleep and alleviate anxiety.

Yet, a cabinet filled with the gifts of nature must be approached with responsibility and respect. Unlike the one-size-fits-all approach typical of pharmaceuticals, natural remedies require us to consider the unique constitution of each individual. Be mindful of potential allergies, interactions with other treatments, and the correct dosages. It's crucial to keep informed and consult with a healthcare advisor when incorporating new remedies into your routine.

Moving beyond the common, there's a wide array of plant-based remedies to explore. Turmeric, with its vibrant golden hue, is lauded for its anti-inflammatory capabilities. Ginger, with its warming qualities, can quell nausea and support digestion. Integrating these elements into your cabinet not only provides direct physical benefits but reinforces the bond between dietary practices and health, illustrating that food truly can be medicine.

Your natural medicine cabinet is not just a compilation of remedies but also a testament to a holistic lifestyle. By choosing natural remedies, you invest in a path of healing that honors both personal well-being and the environment. This journey requires curiosity, learning, and a willingness to engage with your health proactively. It empowers you to take the reins of your wellness, offering alternatives that work gently with your body rather than against it.

Simple, everyday items can also play an essential role in your cabinet. Apple cider vinegar, for example, is known for its antimicrobial properties and can be used as a natural digestive tonic. Similarly, honey is a natural cough suppressant and antibacterial agent. These kitchen staples aren't just good for cooking; they hold a revered place in traditional medicine practices worldwide.

As you cultivate your natural medicine cabinet, embrace the spirit of discovery. Each new addition is an opportunity to learn about its benefits and historical uses. Storytelling has long been at the heart of passing down healing traditions, and by creating a cabinet tailored to your needs, you become a part of this living history, crafting stories of health and healing for future generations.

While the ingredients you gather are important, so are the vessels that hold them. Opt for glass over plastic to store your tinctures and oils, as it reduces the risk of chemical leaching and helps maintain the remedy's integrity. Keep everything clearly labeled to avoid confusion, making sure to note the date of preparation for perishable items, ensuring they are used at their peak potency.

In this endeavor, balance is key. Building a natural medicine cabinet is not about rejecting modern medicine but about complementing it. It's about seeking harmony between conventional and traditional knowledge, a fusion that can enrich our lives with the wisdom of both worlds. With this integration, you're not just embracing a treatment but a philosophy that champions the interconnectedness of life and the art of nurturing it.

Your journey in creating a natural medicine cabinet is as much about exploring internal landscapes as it is about organizing your physical space. With every herb, tincture, and oil, there's a story of healing waiting to unfold—a testament to your commitment to a healthier, more empowered, and connected life. May each element become a catalyst for transformation, nurturing not just your body, but your spirit and the world around you.

In essence, creating a natural medicine cabinet becomes an act of self-care that is deeply aligned with the rhythms of the earth. It's where ancient practices harmonize with modern insights, weaving a tapestry of wellness that is uniquely yours. So gather your supplies, follow where your intuition leads, and let the magic of nature guide you on this transformative path to health and healing.

Addressing Common Household Health Concerns

In today's fast-paced world, it's easy to overlook the small signals our bodies send when something's off. Yet, these very signals often hold the key to fostering a healthier home environment. Addressing common household health concerns doesn't require a vast arsenal of pharmaceuticals but rather a thoughtful approach integrating natural remedies.

Consider the humble cold. Rather than immediately reaching for over-the-counter medications, explore the effectiveness of herbal teas like ginger or elderberry. These infusions have long been celebrated for their immune-boosting properties. A warm cup with a drizzle of honey can soothe a sore throat and provide comfort during chilly evenings.

Headaches, too, are a common woe. Instead of defaulting to painkillers, discover the benefits of peppermint oil. A gentle massage on the temples with a few drops can bring relief, thanks to its cooling and calming properties. Creating a peaceful environment with dimmed lights and quiet can further amplify the effects.

Digestive issues are another area where natural remedies shine. Chamomile tea is a classic choice for relieving bloating and indigestion. Its soothing properties not only help settle the stomach but also promote relaxation, aiding better sleep. Similarly, incorporating ginger in meals can alleviate nausea and enhance digestion.

Muscle aches often follow long days or unexpected strains. Epsom salts are a natural solution that have been used for centuries. A warm bath with Epsom salts can ease tension and relax muscles, making this remedy both nurturing and effective.

Anxiety and stress have unfortunately become commonplace. Here, the mind-body connection plays an important role. Lavender essential oil is renowned for reducing stress. Diffusing it in a cozy corner of your home or applying it topically with a carrier oil can foster a serene atmosphere.

Allergies can be particularly challenging, especially as seasons change. Consider local honey as a sweet ally in combating them. Eating honey that is locally sourced may help the body adapt to local pollen, reducing allergic reactions over time. Although this approach requires patience and consistency, its natural and delicious nature makes it worthwhile.

Skin conditions like eczema or dryness can often be managed with natural means. Coconut oil, rich in moisture and healing properties, can be applied directly to the skin. It acts as a gentle, nourishing barrier that helps lock in hydration. Oatmeal baths are another soothing treatment, providing relief from itching and irritation.

While these remedies offer gentle solutions, it's important to remember that versatility is key. Adapt and experiment with these suggestions to make them personal. Every household and individual is unique, and finding what resonates most with your family's needs can transform everyday challenges into manageable experiences.

Additionally, consider developing a natural medicine cabinet. By stocking it with essential oils, herbal teas, and other holistic essentials, you're better equipped to address common ailments. This preparedness not only fosters independence from pharmaceuticals but also builds confidence in managing health concerns naturally.

Ultimately, addressing common household health concerns with natural remedies enriches the home environment, shifting focus from treating symptoms to nurturing well-being. Inviting nature into our daily rituals encourages a holistic approach that prioritizes balance, mindfulness, and proactive care.

Chapter 10:
The Art of Natural Detoxification

In our journey toward wellness, cleansing the body of accumulated toxins serves as a powerful ally, nurturing both vitality and clarity. With a focus on natural detoxification, we are invited to embrace practices rooted in simplicity and harmony with our environment. Honor your body by integrating thoughtful detox strategies, creating a nurturing space for regeneration. From infusions of lemon and ginger to soothing baths enriched with Epsom salts, these techniques harmonize with your body's innate wisdom. As you incorporate these gentle rituals, remember that detoxification is not just a physical act, but a mindful engagement with your body's rhythms, empowering and inspiring a holistic transformation. Through intentional choices and thoughtful preparation, you enhance your natural healing capacity, supporting a life of balance and renewed energy.

Detox Strategies for Home Use

Natural detoxification doesn't have to be complicated or expensive. Embracing simple strategies at home can significantly enhance your body's ability to cleanse itself effectively. Our bodies are equipped with intrinsic detoxification systems, including the liver, kidneys, and skin. However, in our modern world, these systems often require support to function optimally.

Begin by reconnecting with nature through the air you breathe. Indoor air quality is often overlooked, yet it plays a pivotal role in detoxification. Houseplants such as *snake plants* and *peace lilies* can help purify the air, absorbing toxins emitted from common household items. Regularly airing out your home and avoiding chemical-laden cleaning products are simple ways to enhance the air you breathe, easing the burden on your respiratory system.

Hydration stands as a cornerstone of any effective detox strategy. Water is a universal solvent, and staying well-hydrated supports the kidneys in filtering waste from the blood. Begin your day with a glass of warm lemon water to kickstart the digestive system and support liver function. Herbal teas, such as dandelion or nettle tea, can provide additional detoxifying benefits, acting as gentle diuretics and promoting liver health.

Lifestyle changes foster powerful transformations. Engaging in regular physical activity not only aids in maintaining a healthy weight but also stimulates the lymphatic system and promotes sweating—a natural form of detoxification. Aim for activities that get your blood pumping and your muscles moving, whether it's a brisk walk, yoga, or a dance session in your living room. Even short bursts of exercise can invigorate your body's detox pathways.

Incorporating detoxifying foods into your diet is both beneficial and delicious. Leafy greens, like kale and spinach, support liver function with their high concentrations of chlorophyll and antioxidants. Cruciferous vegetables, such as broccoli and cauliflower, contain compounds that aid in the production of the body's detoxification enzymes. Whole grains, nuts, and seeds offer vital nutrients and fiber, promoting healthy digestion and regularity. Consider making these foods staples in your daily meals.

Fasting or intermittent fasting practices have been revered for centuries as natural methods of detoxification. Allowing the body a break from constant digestion offers it time to divert energy to cellular repair and toxin elimination. Beginners might try a simple overnight fast, extending the time between dinner and breakfast. Listen to your body, understanding that fasting should be gentle and supportive, never extreme or punishing.

An often underestimated detox strategy involves the mind. Stress can impair the body's ability to detoxify, and finding healthy outlets for stress can dramatically improve your detox efforts. Practices such as meditation, journaling, and breathwork can help alleviate the burden of stress. Incorporating mindfulness into your daily routine ensures that your mind and body work in harmony, promoting holistic detoxification.

Cleansing practices extend to the products we choose to put on our bodies. Conventional beauty and personal care products often contain parabens, sulfates, and synthetic fragrances, which can accumulate in the body over time. Switching to natural alternatives can reduce this toxic load. Opt for products with simple, recognizable ingredients, or try making your own using ingredients like coconut oil, shea butter, and essential oils.

In herbal baths, we find both solace and detoxification. Epsom salt baths are renowned for their ability to draw out toxins while replenishing the body's magnesium levels. Add a few drops of eucalyptus or lavender essential oil for an aromatherapeutic boost. The ritual of a bath encourages a pause in daily life, providing a time to unwind and reset.

Seasonal detox routines align with nature's rhythms. As the seasons shift, our bodies often benefit from a corresponding shift in diet and habits. In spring and autumn, a gentle cleanse using lighter meals and increased hydration can prepare the body for the changing weather. Consistent, small daily actions often build towards profound, long-term benefits.

Acknowledge the power of sleep in detoxification. During deep sleep, the brain's glymphatic system works to clear waste products.

Create an environment conducive to restful sleep by maintaining a consistent bedtime, reducing blue light exposure in the evening, and perhaps incorporating calming herbs like chamomile or valerian root tea.

Finally, let's not overlook the social and emotional aspects of detoxification. Surrounding yourself with supportive, health-conscious individuals can provide motivation and accountability. Share meals, recipes, and experiences, creating a community of wellness that uplifts and inspires.

Remember, the journey to natural detoxification is personal and ongoing. Small, sustainable changes yield the most significant impact, nurturing a body that feels alive and vibrant. Embrace the art of detoxing at home, and revel in the newfound vitality it brings.

Recipes and Techniques for Cleansing

In the journey toward personal wellness, cleansing the body is an essential step that fosters balance and restores vitality. Often, the modern lifestyle burdens our systems with toxins from processed foods, pollution, and stress. Fortunately, natural detoxification can support our body's innate ability to purify itself, allowing us to rediscover the state of well-being we were meant to enjoy. This journey to detoxification is a holistic one, respecting the connection between body, mind, and spirit.

To begin with, one of the simplest and most effective techniques is ensuring ample hydration. Water is nature's ultimate cleanser. Drinking sufficient amounts daily aids in flushing out toxins that accumulate in our cells. Try starting each day with a glass of warm lemon water. This simple ritual introduces a gentle, natural acidity that supports the liver's detoxifying functions, stimulates digestion, and encourages an overall sense of rejuvenation. For an added boost, consider infusing your water with slices of cucumber and mint. This not only enhances the flavor but also provides additional antioxidant benefits.

Let's delve into the realm of herbal teas, which are remarkable tools for cleansing. Different teas target different organ systems, offering a variety of benefits. Dandelion root tea is praised for its supportive role in liver detoxification due to its ability to improve bile flow. Meanwhile, nettle tea assists in kidney health and is known for its diuretic properties, helping to remove toxins through increased urine production. When creating your own cleansing tea blend, spend some time understanding each herb and its properties. This mindfulness will ensure that the blend complements your unique constitution and detox goals.

Fiber is another key player in the detox process, as it helps maintain healthy digestion by pushing waste materials through the intestines effectively. Including fiber-rich foods like chia seeds, flaxseeds, and psyllium husk in your diet can be immensely beneficial. You can make a simple cleanse-promoting breakfast by stirring a tablespoon of chia seeds into your favorite nut milk, letting it sit overnight. In the morning, top with fresh fruits and a sprinkle of cinnamon for a balanced start to your day.

Incorporating green smoothies into your daily routine can be transformative. These vibrant drinks are packed with chlorophyll, a powerful detoxifier that can bind to heavy metals and toxins and facilitate their removal from the body. Try a blend of spinach, kale, apple, and ginger. The greens provide essential vitamins and minerals, the apple adds natural sweetness and fiber, while ginger offers anti-inflammatory and digestive benefits. Experiment with different combinations to keep your palate engaged and nutrient intake varied.

Sweating is an often overlooked yet powerful means of detoxification. Our skin is our largest organ, and through sweat, it helps expel toxins. Regular physical activity not only promotes sweating but also stimulates lymphatic circulation, which is crucial for immune function and waste removal. For a more passive approach, consider infrared saunas, which can induce deeper sweating compared to conventional ones. Combined with cold showers, this practice can invigorate circulation and provide a profound sense of cleansing.

Beyond physical practices, reflection through journaling or meditation can initiate emotional cleansing, relieving stress and promoting a balanced outlook on life. Regularly expressing thoughts and emotions on paper or through meditative practice offers mental clarity, which is an essential component of any detox regimen. Perhaps start with a few minutes each day, focusing on mindfulness and gratitude, allowing the mind to declutter just as we seek to do with our bodies.

In the spirit of integrating these techniques seamlessly into your lifestyle, it's important to approach detoxification with flexibility and personal intuition. Adapt these recipes and methods to align with your body's signals and needs. Listen to what your body tells you, as it provides signals about when it requires cleansing or rest.

Transitioning into a practice of natural detoxification should be a nurturing and supportive experience. By empowering yourself with these tools and approaches, you're not just promoting physical health but embracing a comprehensive approach that binds the body, mind, and spirit. Remember, the goal of detoxification isn't just about removal; it's about creating space for renewal and vibrancy.

Chapter 11:
Child-Safe Remedies at Home

In the gentle art of nurturing our children, nature offers a treasure trove of supportive remedies that can ease their discomforts safely and effectively. Understanding which natural ingredients are both potent and gentle enough for a child's delicate system is crucial. A simple chamomile tea can soothe an upset stomach, while a lavender-scented room can ease a restless mind into peaceful slumber. Honey, that golden elixir, not only delights young taste buds but also coats sore throats with its soothing properties—though always remember, it's not for infants under one year. Embracing these natural remedies empowers parents to become healers in their own homes while teaching children to respect and harness nature's bounty. With a focus on safety and simplicity, these remedies offer a path to wellness in which love and care are the primary ingredients, reminding us that sometimes the best medicine is only a pantry away.

Gentle Treatments for Young Ones

Navigating the world of natural remedies for children requires both sensitivity and care. Children, with their tender systems and unique needs, benefit immensely from remedies that are as gentle as they are effective. It's a journey that calls parents to step into a nurturing role, where intuition and knowledge guide decisions. Using natural treatments not only eases common childhood ailments but also instills habits of wellness from a young age, setting the foundation for a lifetime of healthful living.

When children aren't feeling their best, it's crucial to address their discomfort with compassion but also effectiveness. Simple home remedies, often derived from ingredients that you might already have in your pantry, can offer relief in many cases. Chamomile tea, for instance, is a soothing solution not only familiar to many but also incredibly versatile. Known for its calming properties, a mild chamomile infusion can ease tummy troubles and help soothe a fussy child before bed.

For respiratory concerns or mild colds, a honey and lemon mixture can be surprisingly effective. Honey, with its natural antimicrobial properties, not only soothes a scratchy throat but also coats it, providing relief from persistent coughs. However, always remember that honey should only be given to children over one year of age. When mixed with a bit of warm water and freshly squeezed lemon juice, this remedy can offer both comfort and healing.

Earaches, a common childhood complaint, respond well to the warm olive oil remedy. A few drops of warm (not hot) olive oil can alleviate the pain and discomfort associated with ear infections. Olive oil acts as a natural lubricant for the ear and can help relieve pressure. Just ensure that it's not used if there's any suspicion of a punctured eardrum.

Lavender essential oil is another staple in any child-friendly home remedy kit. Known for its calming and soothing properties, lavender oil can be used in a variety of ways. One simple method is to add a drop or two to a child's evening bath, promoting relaxation and deeper sleep. Alternatively, a few drops can be placed in a diffuser to promote a calm ambiance during naptime or an evening wind-down routine.

Gentle physical interventions can also be a part of natural home treatments. A lukewarm sponge bath can be invaluable for alleviating mild fevers. This method not only helps to regulate body temperature but offers a soothing, comforting experience for the child. Remember to avoid cold water, which can cause shivering and possibly raise the body temperature further. It's important that treatments reassure the child and make them feel loved and cared for.

Hydration plays a critical role in a child's recovery from minor illnesses. Encouraging kids to sip on herbal teas, water, or natural fruit-infused beverages can support bodily functions and boost overall recovery. Often, a child may not realize they're dehydrated, but by offering beverages regularly, parents can ensure they maintain adequate fluid intake. This simple yet vital step aids digestion, keeps headaches at bay, and ensures energy levels are maintained.

The art of healing with touch can't be overstated. Gentle massages using light pressure can ease growing pains or stomach discomfort. A blend of coconut oil with a drop of chamomile or lavender oil can be used to massage the child's abdomen in a circular, clockwise motion, aiding digestion and alleviating gas. Massage is a powerful way to deepen parent-child connections while also addressing physical discomfort.

Home environments also play a role in the healing process. A space filled with sunlight and fresh air can work wonders on a child's mood and health. Ensure their play area is well-ventilated and consider using indoor plants to improve air quality. In addition to physical remedies, these environmental considerations can support emotional and physical well-being.

We often underestimate the healing power of sound. Soft music or nature sounds can create a serene environment that aids healing and comfort. Whether it's the gentle notes of a lullaby or the rhythmic sound of ocean waves, finding the right auditory background can significantly enhance a child's rest and recovery.

All these remedies, gentle and nurturing, serve to remind us of the body's natural inclination towards healing. With a bit of knowledge and a lot of love, these simple, home-based solutions can empower parents to deal with everyday health challenges confidently. There's an immense gratification that comes from tapping into nature's resources, knowing that remedying a child's ailment doesn't always necessitate a trip to the pharmacy.

As we engage with these gentle treatments, it's essential to maintain a balance. Always observe how a child responds to any remedy and be ready to seek professional medical advice if something feels beyond your comfort level. Children are resilient, but they also require precise attunement to their needs. By pairing the wisdom of natural remedies with modern knowledge and instincts, you ensure that they receive the gentlest care possible. Each time you offer a remedy, you foster a lifelong connection for them to natural wellness, instilling habits that encourage a balanced, healthy lifestyle.

Precautions and Best Practices

When it comes to using home remedies for children, it's essential to tread carefully. Children are not just small adults; their bodies are still developing, which means they can react differently to various substances, even natural ones. The first rule is simple: less is more. You should always start with the smallest possible dose and observe how your child responds. This approach minimizes the risk of adverse reactions, giving you the peace of mind to explore holistic solutions without compromising safety.

Before diving into any home remedy, it's crucial to understand the basic principle of knowing the source. Ingredients should be fresh, organic, and free from contaminants. Commercially available products can sometimes contain preservatives or other additives that may not be suitable for children. If you're unsure of the purity of an ingredient, don't hesitate to consult a professional or seek out trusted brands that specialize in child-safe products.

Always keep an open line of communication with your child's pediatrician. While you might be enthusiastic about natural treatments, your child's doctor can provide invaluable guidance based on years of training and experience. Be transparent about any remedies you're considering; they can offer advice about potential interactions with medications your child may be taking or other health considerations. Working together with healthcare professionals ensures that you're not navigating these waters alone and that your choices are well-informed.

Allergies are another critical point of consideration. Before applying any new ingredient topically or administering it orally, perform a patch test. Apply a small amount of the substance to your child's forearm and wait 24 hours to monitor for any signs of irritation or adverse reactions. It's a simple but effective step that can prevent discomfort and distress for your little one. Allergic reactions can be particularly acute in children, so this precaution provides an added layer of safety.

It's equally important to create a nurturing environment when administering these remedies. Children are often sensitive to their surroundings. A calm, supportive setting enhances the healing process. This means setting aside specific times for treatment sessions when both you and your child are relaxed and receptive. Trust the process, and allow the therapeutic environment to work synergistically with the chosen remedy.

One shouldn't forget the significance of understanding dosages and frequencies specific to children. You can't simply scale down an adult dosage. Instead, take into consideration the child's weight, age, and specific health needs. Resources like books or reputable online databases specializing in herbal remedies for children can be invaluable. They often provide child-friendly recipes and dosing guidelines that take the guesswork out of the process.

Education is your ally. Equip yourself with knowledge from reliable sources to ensure that every decision has a strong foundation. Join forums with other parents and caregivers who value natural health, and exchange insights about what works and what doesn't. These communities can offer real-world experiences that textbooks might not cover, giving you a broader perspective.

Lastly, be adaptable. Every child is unique, and what works brilliantly for one might not work at all for another. Be willing to adjust methods or try different remedies when necessary. Keep a journal of what you've tried, notes on successes, side effects, and any changes in the child's wellbeing. This ongoing record will serve as a valuable reference as you continue to navigate the journey of natural remedies.

Chapter 12:
Natural Aging and
Longevity Strategies

As we journey through life, the art of aging gracefully becomes not just a priority, but a testament to our understanding and acceptance of natural living. Embracing natural aging involves recognizing the profound wisdom in simplicity and cultivating habits that align our bodies with enduring vitality. Regular movement, nourishing food, and authentic social connections are the keystones of longevity, acting as gentle catalysts that unlock the body's inherent potential for renewal. Here, we delve into time-honored remedies that nurture this process, such as antioxidant-rich herbs and mindfulness practices that combat oxidative stress and nourish the spirit. By integrating these strategies into daily life, we empower ourselves to transition into each subsequent chapter with strength and solace. This holistic path doesn't just extend years but enriches them, rooting us in the present with a vibrant and enduring sense of well-being.

Remedies for Supporting Healthy Aging

As we continue to explore the rich landscape of natural healing, it's essential to discuss remedies that help support healthy aging. Life is a journey of growth and transformation, and with it comes the wisdom of experience. However, it also brings changes to our bodies that require gentle and effective care. Through the thoughtful application of natural remedies, we can support our bodies in maintaining vitality and well-being as the years pass.

The foundation of healthy aging lies in understanding and embracing the power of nature. Let's start with herbs. Herbs are nature's pharmacy; they provide powerful support in aging gracefully. Take turmeric, for instance. With its vibrant color and versatile uses, it's loaded with curcumin, a compound renowned for its anti-inflammatory and antioxidant properties. Studies suggest it may help reduce the impacts of aging on the brain and body.

Ginkgo biloba is another herbal ally. Long celebrated in traditional medicine, it may enhance circulation, particularly to the brain. This can boost cognitive function, helping to keep your memory sharp. While science is still delving into its full effects, anecdotal evidence from across cultures speaks volumes about its benefits.

Let's not overlook the importance of everyday movement. Regular physical activity doesn't just keep the muscles and joints flexible; it also supports heart health and mental clarity. Options like yoga and tai chi are worth considering, offering low-impact exercise that can improve balance, flexibility, and overall coordination. They also bring an element of mindfulness, helping the mind stay as nimble as the body.

Nutrition plays a pivotal role in how our bodies age. A diet rich in fruits, vegetables, whole grains, and lean proteins can provide essential nutrients and antioxidants that fight free radicals. Berries, with their high levels of antioxidants, are particularly beneficial. Foods like fish, rich in omega-3 fatty acids, support brain and heart health. These nutrients are critical as we age and strive for longevity.

Hydration is another key part of the puzzle. As we age, our sense of thirst may diminish, making it imperative to consciously maintain adequate fluid intake. Water promotes cellular health and keeps skin looking youthful. Herbal teas can be both hydrating and offer additional benefits, like chamomile for its calming properties or green tea for its catechins.

Elara Greenwood

Don't underestimate the mind-body connection in the aging process. Techniques like meditation can foster mental clarity and emotional resilience. Regular meditation practice has been linked to increased gray matter density in the brain, which could slow the brain's aging process. Even a few minutes daily can provide profound benefits for mental and emotional health.

Social connections are integral to healthy aging. Engaging with a community, whether through family, friends, or social groups, can combat feelings of loneliness and depression, significantly impacting longevity and quality of life. These interactions stimulate mental engagement and provide emotional support, crucial factors in maintaining overall health.

Natural supplements can also play a role, though it's important to choose them wisely. Options like Coenzyme Q10 (CoQ10) and omega-3 supplements could offer support for heart health and cognitive function. It's crucial, however, to consult with a healthcare provider to ensure these supplements complement your health needs and existing conditions.

Beyond the physical, embracing a sense of purpose is vital. Having goals and passions keeps the spirit lively, providing drive and direction. Whether through volunteer work, hobbies, or lifelong learning, staying engaged in activities that bring joy and fulfillment is essential for a vibrant life.

Recognizing the importance of rest and sleep is equally vital. Our bodies repair and rejuvenate during sleep, making quality rest a cornerstone of health. Herbal remedies like valerian root or lavender can aid sleep naturally, without the need for heavy pharmaceuticals.

Finally, consider integrating uplifting practices like laughter and gratitude into everyday life. Both have been shown to release endorphins, reduce stress, and improve overall mood. Maintaining a positive outlook can foster resilience and strength as we navigate the practicalities of aging.

There's no one-size-fits-all approach to aging, but these steps highlight the potential of natural remedies to provide a supportive framework. With diligence and care, we can embrace each year as a promise of new opportunities for growth and learning. Through connecting with nature, our communities, and ourselves, we empower not only our own lives but become beacons of healthy aging for others.

Embracing a Holistic Approach to Longevity

In today's fast-paced world, where every tick of the clock seems to push us towards a future replete with uncertainties and challenges, the pursuit of longevity has emerged as a profound endeavor. It's about more than simply prolonging life; it's about enriching those extra years with vitality and purpose. Embracing a holistic approach isn't just a path—it's a transformation inviting us to reconnect with age-old wisdom while harmonizing it with contemporary insights.

Living a long, robust life doesn't solely hinge on genetics or the latest scientific breakthroughs. At its core, it involves a deep and meaningful connection to every aspect of our being: the body, mind, and spirit. A holistic approach acknowledges this intricate interplay, fostering an awareness that every choice we make—what we eat, how we move, how we think—influences our well-being. Here, wisdom becomes the compass, guiding us toward balanced living.

Nutrition stands as a crucial pillar in this holistic paradigm. Moving beyond mere calorie counting, it's about nourishing our bodies with foods that are as close to their natural state as possible. Whole grains, fresh fruits, and vibrant vegetables become more than just ingredients; they are the elixirs sustaining our vitality. Consider integrating colorful, antioxidant-rich berries into your diet. They're small but mighty allies in the battle against oxidative stress, a key player in aging.

Physical activity, too, dances alongside nutrition, forming a dynamic duo in our quest for longevity. Gone are the days when exercise was reserved for the young or the intensely athletic. Embracing movement that suits our preferences and physical capabilities, be it a gentle yoga flow or a brisk nature walk, is fundamental. Our bodies are meant to move, and when they do, they release endorphins—the body's natural mood elevators and painkillers—infusing our days with energy and joy.

However, a holistic approach doesn't stop at the physical. It's equally about tending to the fertile grounds of our minds. Stress, an inevitable component of modern life, can become a corrosive force when unchecked. Techniques like mindfulness and meditation are not just trends—they're ancient practices that have anchored humanity through the ages. By quieting the mind's chatter, they create space for clarity and serenity, reducing stress and enhancing our mental resilience.

Spirituality, too, deserves its place in this mosaic of well-being. It's not necessarily about religion but about nurturing a connection to something greater than ourselves. It might be found in the awe of nature, in acts of kindness, or in moments of introspection where we reflect on our life's purpose. This sense of belonging and meaning can become an inner compass, providing solace and direction amidst life's ebbs and flows.

Social connections are another essential thread in the fabric of holistic longevity. Humans are inherently social creatures, and our relationships—be they with family, friends, or the broader community—have a profound influence on our health. Who can deny the warmth of companionship, the comfort of a shared smile, or the resilience born from communal support? These interactions nourish our souls, making them as vital as the food we eat or the air we breathe.

A crucial aspect of this holistic strategy is the recognition of the subtle but profound rhythms of life. Engaging with the natural cycles of day and night—honoring our innate circadian rhythms—ensures we recharge and rejuvenate optimally. Practices like ensuring ample sunlight exposure during the day and cultivating a serene environment for sleep at night can synchronize our inner clocks, promoting restorative rest.

Of course, embracing a holistic approach to longevity isn't without its challenges. It's easy to become overwhelmed in a world where information is abundant yet often contradictory. Choosing which advice to follow or which lifestyle to adopt requires discerning wisdom. This is where personal intuition, guided by research and understanding, becomes invaluable. The journey is uniquely individual, requiring that we listen to our bodies and hearts.

As we traverse the path of holistic aging, we're reminded that this isn't a solo journey. We carry with us the knowledge of generations past, updated by the insights of present-day thinkers and doers. Together, they form a rich tapestry of guidance informing our daily choices—not as restrictions but as liberations from unfound fear and doubt.

Finally, let's not ignore the power of laughter and joy. These intangible elements can soften life's challenges, etching moments of happiness into our being. A positive outlook, despite life's inevitable adversities, can be a fountain of youth all its own. The very act of seeing beauty in the mundane, of expressing gratitude for the present and hope for the future, can transform the ordinary into extraordinary

In conclusion, embracing a holistic approach to longevity is more than a mere tactic or strategy—it's a way of life that respects and honors the totality of human experience. By aligning mind, body, and spirit, and acknowledging our connection to the world around us, we not only aim to live longer but to live better. This integration doesn't promise to make life devoid of struggles but equips us with the resilience and grace to meet them.

As we continue on this path, our focus should remain steadfast on the journey rather than the destination. The small, deliberate changes we make today can lead to a more fulfilling tomorrow, ensuring our twilight years are not just years added to life but life added to years. Through this holistic lens, we find not just the key to a longer life but the secret to a richer, more meaningful existence.

Conclusion

The journey through the many chapters of this exploration into natural healing and wellness has illuminated the power and accessibility of home-based remedies. We've wandered along paths once trodden by ancient healers and explored how these age-old traditions dovetail with modern insights, painting a comprehensive picture of our relationship with nature's bounty. This isn't just a tapestry of methods and solutions; it's a call to embrace a lifestyle that prioritizes balance, sustainability, and self-care.

Our exploration began by delving into the origins of natural healing, laying the foundation for everything we've discussed. This was more than a theoretical exercise; it was an invitation to reconnect with a legacy that spans generations, reminding us that healing isn't a recent innovation but an ancient art. This understanding enhances our appreciation of herbal medicine, which you now know not only as a therapeutic tool but also as a medium that empowers you to take charge of your well-being. Through growing and harvesting your own herbs, you strengthen this connection, nurturing both body and earth.

Essential oils and aromatherapy offered another realm of possibilities, proving that healing can also be joyful and sensory. By crafting your own blends, you've learned a skill that is as much about creativity as it is about science. It's a gentle reminder that healing is as much about the journey as it is about the destination. Similarly, the role of nutrition in health is critical and transformative. By adopting dietary principles that foster natural health, you're not merely avoiding ailments; you're laying the groundwork for vibrant living. Food becomes medicine, lots of nature's pharmacy.

Homeopathy and supplements widened our scope by introducing customizable solutions to common ailments. These aren't just alternatives; they're proactive steps towards health that reflect a deep understanding of individual needs. Whether it's choosing quality supplements or preparing homeopathic treatments, what's clear is the importance of informed choices. This theme of empowerment is further reinforced when we acknowledge how the mind and body are inherently linked. Techniques that nurture both are integral to attaining a harmonious state of well-being.

When it comes to skin care and household remedies, the message is one of simplicity and efficacy. These everyday solutions testify to the versatility of natural components and their capacity to care for us from the inside out. They encourage us to be mindful of what we apply to our bodies and the spaces we inhabit, extending the philosophy of holistic care to every part of our lives.

The art of detoxification unveils methods that can purify and rejuvenate without harsh chemicals or strenuous protocols. By focusing on gentler regimes, we align ourselves with rhythms that honor our bodies' capabilities. Such detox strategies are not just about elimination; they're about transformation, paving the way for renewed vitality.

Our youngest loved ones benefit as well from gentle and child-safe remedies. These treatments affirm that natural healing is a family affair, one that can be passed seamlessly from generation to generation. Ensuring that our practices respect their delicate systems is a testament to the careful thought woven throughout this guide. As for the journey of aging, we've touched upon techniques and perspectives that underscore aging not as a decline, but a transition—a stage where nature supports an active, vibrant life.

In wrapping up this exploration, it's clear that the pursuit of natural healing is deeply personal and profoundly communal. Every remedy, solution, and strategy discussed reflects a broader commitment to wellness—one that doesn't exist in isolation but is enhanced by the collective wisdom of those who came before us. Through this framework, you are not just a passive recipient of these ideas; you are an active participant in the healing dance between nature and humanity.

Ultimately, this book is an invitation to trust in nature's immense potential, as well as in your innate ability to harness it. With knowledge comes the power to make informed choices that favor wellness over dependency. It's about choice: opting for remedies that are not quick fixes, but rather, contributors to sustained health. May you carry forward the practices and philosophies you've discovered here, using them to chart a path unique to you, one that truly embodies natural healing in every sense.

Appendix A:
Resources and Further Reading

As we journey through the world of natural healing, it's important to remember that the art of self-care is both timeless and evolving. Armed with knowledge and a willingness to explore, you can deepen your understanding and enrich your practice of home-based health solutions. Here, we've curated a selection of resources that will support your ongoing exploration and provide further insight into the diverse and holistic world of natural remedies.

Books and Publications

- *Healing with Whole Foods: Asian Traditions and Modern Nutrition* by Paul Pitchford - A comprehensive guide on balancing physical, emotional, and spiritual health through nutrition.

- *The Complete Book of Essential Oils and Aromatherapy* by Valerie Ann Worwood - A must-read for those eager to delve deeper into the benefits and uses of essential oils.

- *The Herbal Medicine-Maker's Handbook: A Home Manual* by James Green - Perfect for beginners and seasoned herbalists who wish to craft their own remedies.

- *The Mindbody Prescription: Healing the Body, Healing the Pain* by John E. Sarno - This book explores the powerful connection between mind and body and how our emotions can affect physical health.

Online Resources

- **National Center for Complementary and Integrative Health (NCCIH)** - Access a wealth of information on various complementary health practices and ongoing research.

- **American Herbalists Guild (AHG)** - An excellent resource for those interested in the practice of herbalism, offering educational resources and professional guidance.

- **Aromatherapy Research and Education (AIRE)** - Stay updated on the latest research and best practices in the field of aromatherapy.

Workshops and Courses

- **Herbal Academy** - Offers a wide array of courses from beginner to advanced levels, suitable for anyone interested in herbal studies.

- **Essential Oil Academy** - Gain practical knowledge through online courses focusing on the safe and effective use of essential oils.

- **Meditation and Mindfulness Centers** - Explore local or online classes and workshops to deepen your understanding of mind-body techniques.

Communities and Forums

- **HerbMentor Forum** - Join a community of herbal enthusiasts to share experiences, seek advice, and learn collectively.

- **Facebook Groups and Online Communities** - Engage with groups dedicated to natural healing topics, such as herbal remedies, essential oils, and homeopathy, for real-life advice and discussions.

In the pursuit of natural health, continual learning is key. Embrace these resources as stepping stones on your path to a balanced life where wellness is crafted through nature and nurturing practices. May these pointers ignite your curiosity, inspire ongoing exploration, and deepen your commitment to nurturing your well-being naturally.